10

Steps to
Better
Living
with Diabetes

Ginger Kanzer-Lewis, RN, BC, EdM, CDE

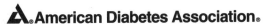

American Diabetes Association®

Cure • Care • Commitment®

Managing Editor, Book Publishing, Abe Ogden; *Acquisitions Editor, Consumer Books,* Robert Anthony; *Editor,* Greg Guthrie; *Production Manager,* Melissa Sprott; *Composition,* Circle Graphics; *Cover Design,* VC Graphics; *Printer,* Data Reproductions Corporation.

Printed in the United States of America
1 3 5 7 9 10 8 6 4 2

The suggestions and information contained in this publication are generally consistent with the *Clinical Practice Recommendations* and other policies of the American Diabetes Association, but they do not represent the policy or position of the Association or any of its boards or committees. Reasonable steps have been taken to ensure the accuracy of the information presented. However, the American Diabetes Association cannot ensure the safety or efficacy of any product or service described in this publication. Individuals are advised to consult a physician or other appropriate health care professional before undertaking any diet or exercise program or taking any medication referred to in this publication. Professionals must use and apply their own professional judgment, experience, and training and should not rely solely on the information contained in this publication before prescribing any diet, exercise, or medication. The American Diabetes Association—its officers, directors, employees, volunteers, and members—assumes no responsibility or liability for personal or other injury, loss, or damage that may result from the suggestions or information in this publication.

∞ The paper in this publication meets the requirements of the ANSI Standard Z39.48-1992 (permanence of paper).

ADA titles may be purchased for business or promotional use or for special sales. To purchase more than 50 copies of this book at a discount, or for custom editions of this book with your logo, contact Lee Romano Sequeira, Special Sales & Promotions, at the address below, or at LRomano@diabetes.org.

For all other inquiries, please call 1-800-DIABETES.

American Diabetes Association
1701 North Beauregard Street
Alexandria, Virginia 22311

Library of Congress Cataloging-in-Publication Data

Kanzer-Lewis, Ginger, 1944-
  10 steps to better living with diabetes / Ginger Kanzer-Lewis.
    p. cm.
  Includes bibliographical references and index.
  ISBN 978-1-58040-259-0 (alk. paper)
  1. Diabetes—Popular works. I. Title. II. Title: Ten steps to better living with diabetes.

RC660.4.K36 2007
616.4'62—dc22
                2007005886

For my husband, Jack, who tells everyone that he's taught me everything I know. I'm not sure about that, but he has taught me about love, courage, and what we can do together. This is our book.

Contents

Foreword

For 30 years, Ginger Kanzer-Lewis has worked with people with diabetes. She has felt and dealt with all of the emotions and challenges that are part of daily life with a chronic disease. Ginger's hands-on experience in helping people live successfully with diabetes has given her the unique perspective from which to write this book. It is a must-read handbook for all people with diabetes, their families, and their friends. I like to think of this book as Ginger's personal letter to every individual with diabetes, providing the information, tools, letters, and other helpful tips that will assist in making a difference in a life with diabetes.

In these pages, you will find ten of the most discussed topics in diabetes self-care. Ginger's practical, no-nonsense information and tips will give you a framework for building a better life with diabetes. Now, not all of these tips apply to everyone, and they're not guaranteed to work because everyone is different, but you will have the options and choices you need to make a positive difference. I am sure that any reader will find something in this book to use to make positive change a real, achievable possibility.

Ginger's wealth of knowledge and experience with diabetes is her true gift, and one that she generously passes along through this book. By reading it, you're giving a gift to yourself. So let Ginger give you a lesson in diabetes education and self-care and read these *10 Steps to Better Living with Diabetes*.

Karmeen Kulkarni
MS, RD, BC-ADM, CDE
President, Health Care & Education
American Diabetes Association, 2005–2006

Acknowledgments

I would like to acknowledge with sincere gratitude all of the people who have made my career a joy and a gift. I have learned from every patient I have ever met and treasure all of the educators who care for people with diabetes. I am grateful to my colleagues, who work day in and day out to give of themselves in our fight to make diabetes a thing of the past.

I would like to thank all the officers, board members, and staff of the American Association of Diabetes Educators, who I believe have encouraged me to reach for new achievements and goals.

I am grateful to the wonderful professionals at the American Diabetes Association who have allowed me to share my thoughts and put up with my stories and rambling. Special thanks go to my editor, Greg Guthrie, who carried me by hand through the editing process of this book.

Lastly, I would like to thank my family for their endless support. I love you all.

Introduction

Welcome. For over 30 years I have taught people with diabetes and have lived with their anger, frustration, stress, and fear, much of it arising from lack of support. I have also watched people with diabetes take their lives back from the disease and make the transition from being a diabetic to being a person who just happens to have diabetes. There have been wonderful developments made in diabetes care, including the invention of incredible new equipment and the development of amazing medications. I have taken part in the advent and success of the diabetes educator and diabetes education. There is potential for great success in the field of diabetes care.

Today, every person with diabetes can reasonably expect to live a long and fairly normal life. I use the word "fairly" because no matter how we have evolved, it is not normal to have to worry about a chronic disease every day and it sure isn't normal to stick yourself with sharp pins. But for now you're going to have to stick your fingers and test your blood, so there's no point in wondering what life would be like if you didn't have to. Now let's get to the good stuff and talk about how you can take control of your life and do the very best that you can.

Consider this book as a personal letter to you or as a face-to-face meeting with your own personal certified diabetes educator. I know, this book is very long, but that's because I like to talk a lot. And I can talk even longer about diabetes. Please remember, though, that I am talking directly to you because I want to help. You can take what you choose from this book and make your own decisions about what will help you manage your diabetes best. Go ahead and read it all or just read the parts that you need right away. You will find some tools and letters in the different chapters that may help you on the way. Feel free to copy those tools and letters and use them in any way that will make your life easier or better. Use anything that you find to be helpful and share it with your friends and family.

If I could, I would talk to everyone everywhere who had diabetes or who took care of people with diabetes. I would talk about the successes we have had in the past few years and how exciting it is to be a part of such great advances. Unfortunately, I can't talk to the entire world, so the next best thing is for me to talk to all of the people whose lives are touched by diabetes through this book. I want to cheer you on and give you hope for a good and healthy future.

Will it take work, a commitment to take control of your diabetes, and a full partnership with your health care professionals to ensure a fine future life? Absolutely! I, and any other diabetes professional, would love to be part of that partnership.

This book is written to help you take control of your life. There are 10 steps that I believe will help you live a better life. Are they guaranteed to absolutely work? Of course not. These are simple steps that you can choose to take, maybe one or two or maybe all of them, but any one of them can definitely get you on the track to better living with diabetes. After all, life is about choices and so is diabetes.

But before we get into all the details, let me tell you a little about myself. My name is Ginger Kanzer-Lewis, and I have the following degrees: RN, BC, EdM, and CDE. These initials stand for Registered Nurse (RN), Board Certified in Staff Development and Continuing Education (BC), Master's Degree in Education (Harvard University) (EdM), and Certified Diabetes Educator (CDE).

I have been a nurse for 40 years, and since 1972, I have been teaching people with diabetes how to take care of themselves. I have been a Director of Education in hospitals all over the northeastern U.S., and I have established programs for health care professionals and taught them how to teach patients, not just about diabetes, but about all kinds of health care issues. A long time ago, I decided that I could help more people if I taught professionals how to better care for and teach patients. As a consultant, I worked at the Joslin clinic in Boston from 1980 to 1994 teaching people to teach. In 2000, I was honored to be the President of the American Association of Diabetes Educators. In 2003, I wrote a book for professionals: *Patient Education: You Can Do It!* That's why I am qualified to help you. I have taught thousands of patients, and countless professional colleagues have attended my programs. While I taught them, they also taught me, and I want to share a lot of these lessons with you. I really think I can help, and I will, if you let me.

Take care,
Ginger Kanzer-Lewis

One

So You Have Diabetes

So you have diabetes. Did you just find out or have you had it for a while and finally decided to do something about it? Don't worry; you are not alone. This is the world I live and work in, and I have the knowledge and experience to give you a tour of the ins and outs of diabetes. There are lots of us here who can help you and who have experiences much like yours: people who have diabetes and professionals who take care of people with diabetes. It is like a diabetes community because each of us has specific roles and each of us deals with diabetes in our own fashion, some better than others.

Not only do I work with people who have diabetes, but I have pre-diabetes myself, so I think about it all the time. My husband has type 2 diabetes, so I am also the spouse of someone with diabetes. If you didn't know it already, your significant others play a major part in living well with diabetes. We will talk to your significant others and about them in this chapter.

DEALING WITH DIAGNOSIS

Are you angry, upset, or confused? You may be frightened, and you may be so worried that you are not sure who to

1

Diabetes Is a Family Affair

Joe Solowiejczyk, a diabetes counselor, once told me that the people who live with people with diabetes should be considered as having their own unique form of diabetes, something that he'd like to call type 3 diabetes. Don't worry! Diabetes isn't contagious.

According to Joe, the loved ones of people with diabetes expend almost as much time and energy on diabetes as the people who have it themselves and are not often given any support or acknowledgment at all. They are as concerned as the patients and are often the ones who have to take it upon themselves to bring healthy cooking into the daily meals, nag them to test their blood sugar levels, make sure all medications are taken at the proper time, or monitor the disease process for complications. Obviously, any loved one could feel overwhelmed and sometimes angry in this situation, feeling that they have taken on a huge burden and have suddenly been tossed into the diabetes community without asking.

talk to or who to tell. You may feel like you want to hit something or just sit alone someplace and cry. That is OK. If you want to scream, go sit in the car and do it, but close the windows. That way, you'll have some privacy and no one will call the police. Please remember, though, that communication is one of the most important parts of your life right now. If you are angry or upset, tell someone that this is how you are feeling and to let you get through it your way. You need to warn people that you are going through a difficult time in your life and that you will include them when you are ready. You don't need to let it all out right away, but you need to keep open the channels of communication. Remember, the people who love you may become frightened and imagine something much worse than diabetes if you don't tell them anything. At this moment, it is OK to say, "I just don't want to talk about it right now."

I know, it stinks having diabetes and it's not fair that you have diabetes. You may just wish that it would go away. You probably have all of these emotions and wonder how you are going to get through this. Unfortunately, there's a hard truth in this situation: your diabetes is not going away. You will have to deal with it. I am sorry. People with diabetes have told me that they don't want to have diabetes. That kind of thinking is normal and part of the process of acceptance, but over the long run, it won't make your life with diabetes any better. I'd like to be taller, but I haven't grown an inch in years. Diabetes won't go away—it's part of you now. As much as I'd love to, I can't make it go away; there is no magic wand in my briefcase or in any health care professional's briefcase or even in his or her office! Maybe a cure will happen someday, but not right now. For a long time, many of us have worked toward the day when a cure is discovered, but we are not there yet. You may see it happen, though. I would love to be there with you, but I'd probably talk your ear off, too.

Keep an eye out for boxes with this DT logo. It stands for "Diabetes Tip," and they're all over this book. Inside them you'll find the little bits of knowledge and wisdom that I've accumulated through my years of working with people with diabetes. I want to share them with you, and maybe you'll find that some of these tips will give you a little boost to better living with diabetes.

The important thing is that you don't have to deal with it alone and that there are over 20 million people in the U.S. in the same boat. Over 6 million of those people don't even know that they have diabetes. Many people have diabetes for about 8 years before it is diagnosed, and sometimes they have already developed complications. In many cases, it is

It Takes a Team

Diabetes is serious, and it needs to be treated aggressively and with a whole team of health care professionals. Throughout this book, I will be talking a lot about PCPs. PCPs are primary care providers, and they're the people who take care of you. A PCP can be your physician (doctor), nurse practitioner, or physician assistant. I will talk about your relationships with all of the people in your life later, but for now let's focus on you and the fact that you have diabetes.

when a person starts having strange symptoms that they go to the doctor and find out that they have diabetes.

REACTING TO DIABETES

Everyone reacts differently when they hear that they have diabetes. Strangely enough, people normally don't panic or become filled with fear when they are diagnosed with diabetes. It's as if diabetes is somehow different from being diagnosed with a disease like cancer or being told that they need to have open-heart surgery. This is not a healthy reaction. I have never met a person who, when told that they have cancer or need heart surgery, said, "That's OK, I'll be fine, and I've been expecting it." Thinking like this scares me. Diabetes can lead to conditions that kill people, so it's no less serious than cancer or a stroke or a heart attack. Remember, diabetes is serious business.

"Diabetes Is in My Family"

Sometimes, I'll talk to patients who recently learned that they have diabetes, and they'll say something like "It's all over my family, so I'm not surprised." If you come from a "diabetic family," then you should be aware of the symptoms and take action. Please don't just accept diabetes as your fate. This is not a helpful reaction to your diagnosis. When you learn you have diabetes, you need to *react*, not just shrug your shoulders and say, "Oh well." You can even start crying or yell at me, that's OK. I'd prefer that, but just saying that you've seen it coming tends to make me really mad.

For people who have lived with diabetes in their families and seen its dangerous consequences and complications, the period surrounding the diagnosis of diabetes is both difficult and complex. It seems to me that people want to avoid dealing with the diabetes that has ravaged their family members and loved ones because it is so absolutely scary. I understand this, and it is true: diabetes is difficult and has serious side effects and complications. What you need to realize, though, is that things are so much better now than when your Aunt Sarah or Uncle Bob had it and lost her or his leg or when even my own grandmother died in what they used to call "insulin shock." If you have diabetes in your family, don't concentrate on the terrible things you've heard and seen. Instead, know that there have been incredible advances in the care and treatment of diabetes over the past 5 years. In fact, there have been so many changes that it's nearly impossi-

I suggest that all people with diabetes have at least one consultation visit with an endocrinologist. This specialist really knows the state-of-the-art treatment in diabetes care and will set a plan of action that you and your primary care provider can confidently follow. Even if you are very comfortable with and confident in your physician, you might want to discuss this. An endocrinologist should see people with complicated diabetes treatments and diabetes complications.

ble for us health care professionals to keep our knowledge and skills up to date!

So let's forget the stories and the past and concentrate on what is current and where the future is going. I am asking you to get your advice about diabetes from health care professionals and not lay magazines and the gossip group. Throughout this book, I will talk about reliable places to get information and send you to safe, bright, and knowledgeable sources for all kinds of help. Sometimes a little bit of the wrong information can be very dangerous. Your friends might call with really exciting information they see on the news and think you should start a certain medication or treatment that they know will cure diabetes. Remember, just because something appears on TV or in the papers does not mean that it is scientifically factual or safe. If you see something interesting, please discuss it with your health care team (see page 17).

Accepting Diabetes in Stages

People may respond differently to being diagnosed with diabetes, but they seem to go through the same stages as people who are told that they are dying. This is normal. Grief is the same whenever it happens, and whether it is fear for your life or a major change in your life, it is still grief. In her book, *On Death and Dying*, Elisabeth Kübler-Ross identified five stages of grief. Let's take diabetes and see how it fits into this scale.

Stage One: Denial and Isolation

Does any of this sound familiar?

- "This is stupid and ridiculous. It can't be happening to me."
- "The lab must have made a mistake. This can't be right. I feel fine, and this is wrong. I won't tell any-

> body, and I'll wait awhile and go back to the doctor
> and get more tests that will come back fine. I must
> have the flu or a urinary tract infection that makes
> me pee all the time."
> - "What does this doctor know? He's not a specialist. I'll
>   go to a different hospital, and they'll say he's wrong.
>   That's what I'll do."

I believe Dr. Kübler-Ross should have called this denial and guilt instead of denial and isolation. It is easy to just ignore things and hope that they will go away, but doing so makes you feel guilty for ignoring it. Then you lie there at three in the morning, when no one else can hear you, and talk to yourself about how maybe you really have to think about this. It seems like a vicious circle.

In their book, *Diabetes Myths, Misconceptions, and Big Fat Lies!*, Kris Swenson and Betty Brackenridge talk about the myths surrounding a new diagnosis. Don't blame yourself. You did not cause this to happen, and eating too many sweets doesn't give you diabetes. You will be astonished how many people will ask you if you are a big sweets or candy eater. As if you ate your way to diabetes through the cookie jar. That's nonsense!

We will talk more about the process later but guilt doesn't make sense. If you can, be honest with yourself. It may take some time. The doctor didn't make a mistake in diagnosing you, and it is true that you have diabetes. This is especially hard for the parents of children who have just been diagnosed with diabetes. They go through terrible feelings of anxiety and guilt, and their process is sometimes so painful that they spend years spoiling the child to try and make up for "giving them diabetes." You can't give anyone diabetes, and no one gave it to you. It does tend to run in families, but it is not inherited.

Take a sharp look at yourself. Are you in this stage? I think that if you are reading this book, then it's quite likely that you have passed this stage. If you were in denial, you

Joannie's Story

The denial stage can be very quick or very prolonged. I have a friend who decided that she was not going to deal with diabetes. She wouldn't talk to me about it because if she did, then she would have to admit to herself that she really had diabetes. She would take the pills the doctor gave her because that was all right and not painful or stressful. She would watch the sweets she ate and try to watch her weight, but she wasn't very serious about it. I tried to give her a glucose meter once, and she politely took it, but hid it in the closet and never used it. She was very determined not to be a diabetic.

Several years later, she had a retinal bleed in one eye and lost part of her vision. She became so frightened that she knew she could not deny having diabetes any longer. We worked together for a long time, and she met with another diabetes educator near her home. She lost weight, started exercising on a regular basis, and improved her diabetes care and her general health. Unfortunately, she had a heart attack several years later, but thankfully she survived. She and her doctor both believed that she survived because she had taken control of her diabetes and gotten her weight, blood pressure, blood sugar, and general health care status under control. Now, several years later, she is doing very well. She helps teach diabetes classes and runs support groups in her community center.

As you can see from this story, denying that you have diabetes—sometimes for years—can result in the development of very serious complications. These complications can be prevented with early treatment, but by avoiding diabetes, the complications only grow worse. Is avoiding the fact that you have diabetes, like in Joannie's case, worth losing your eyesight?

would have walked right by the diabetes section of the bookstore. Instead, you are getting help and taking steps to make your life better. That's great. Still, to better understand these steps, think back to when you were diagnosed with diabetes. How did you handle it? Is that moment clear and cold in your memory? Did you say, "Not me. I don't believe this"?

Sometimes it just helps to set a deadline for not believing in or dealing with diabetes right after diagnosis. Tell yourself, "I won't believe this now, but I will think about it right after the weekend." Remember, though, to make sure that you don't put the thought of diabetes so far away that it can't ever come out. That *is* denial.

In many cases, even if you are still having trouble accepting that you have diabetes, it may be worthwhile to try some role playing instead. Try this. Let's say a friend or family member was just diagnosed with diabetes. What would you say to him or her to help relieve the shock of this diagnosis? Maybe talking to someone else with diabetes about their diagnosis would be helpful. Sometimes, facts help people move past denial, so ask to see the form with the laboratory work and the results of the tests. Ask the doctor for the diagnosis criteria that show what these test results actually mean. Maybe a list of the symptoms of diabetes would help. This would give you a chance to compare the present symptoms with those in the list. Do these symptoms apply to your imagined friend or family member? Do they apply to you? Sometimes, it really helps to face the facts when they are written down.

Second Stage: Anger

Does any of this sound familiar?
- "Why me?"
- "I don't deserve this."

> ■ "This isn't fair."
> ■ "There are bad people in the world: drug dealers and murderers and very horrible people. Let them get diabetes, but not me. I am a good person."

Get mad. It's OK, but sometime, you'll have to move past it. You know when you are angry. How do you show it? Do you scream at everyone? Do you throw things? Do you cry? Do you hide your feelings? Take out a piece a paper and write down what you do when you are really angry.

Have you done any of the things on your list lately? Do you snap at people more than you used to? Have you stopped enjoying the things that used to be fun? These can be signs of anger or depression (more on that later). Have you told your significant other that you are really angry that this is happening to you? What did you say to your health care providers when they told you that you had diabetes?

If you can't seem to shake off this anger, talk to a professional. I like to recommend Harold S. Kushner's wonderful book, *When Bad Things Happen to Good People*, for people who are coping with anger at being diagnosed with diabetes. Often, people are relieved when I tell them that it is all right and normal to be angry. You may find that the anger returns from time to time during your lifetime, when you are reminded that diabetes will not go away and that it will require a lifetime commitment. Remember, if the anger doesn't get in the way of your own personal health, if it does not get in the way of your diabetes care, then you have permission to be ticked off. Anger is normal, and it's human. It's OK. I give you permission to be angry. Now, does that feel better?

Don't hold on to your anger for so long that you cannot move forward. Some people hold on to the anger and then, because they're so angry, they don't do anything to care for themselves. If you keep this anger going and avoid starting treatment and getting your blood sugar under control, then you put yourself in jeopardy of developing the complications that can be avoided.

Third Stage: Bargaining

Does any of this sound familiar?

- "I know what I'll do. I'll go on a diet. I can exercise. That'll be easy! Maybe if I do all of this, then that diabetes thing will go away."
- "If I pray more or go to church more often, God will take this problem away."
- "I'll take all of my medications, and eventually, my blood sugar will be so good that I won't have to worry about diabetes ever again."
- "If only I had listened to my doctor and taken my medicine."

Does any of this sound familiar? Does it sound like something you have ever said? What kinds of bargains have you made with yourself or a higher power? I respect whatever beliefs you have and honor them, but sometimes prayers don't get answered. You don't have the time to sit around and wait. There are lots of people asking for help. You need to help yourself. You can negotiate all you want, but diabetes is not going away. Diabetes can be controlled and be effectively dealt with, but it cannot be cured.

A patient once told me that she knew she should go to church more often and that if she did, then God would make her diabetes go away, like a cold. I have another patient who is convinced that if he just loses enough weight and never eats "sweets" again, then it will go away and he can stop sticking his fingers and taking those "damn" pills. He's a brilliant man and knows all about diabetes, but he is not willing to give up the idea that he can fix it. I'm still working with him. His blood sugars are coming down, and he sees a doctor regularly now. He still gets angry when I remind him that he will have to deal with diabetes for the rest of his life, but if it stirs him up to take better control of himself, then I don't care. He's my patient, and I will not give up on him.

I think that you can make a bargain with yourself, but it has to be productive. I like to think of productive bargains as contracts you make with yourself to take better care of your diabetes. In this sense, you're setting goals and deciding which benchmarks you will set to make achieving these goals possible. Maybe you're even setting what your rewards will be when you reach your goals.

I do this myself and set new goals often. For example, as an educator I am willing to teach you how to manage your meals. Your part of the bargain/contract is that you will keep a record of everything you eat for three days. This is a productive bargain because it sets goals and provides a cooperative way for us both to achieve them. I am not really bargaining with you, unless I say something like "I will teach you about your medications; that way, you might know to take them every day and your diabetes will get better." That's unproductive because I'm not giving you the tools to succeed. When you think about caring for your diabetes, make sure that you give yourself the tools to succeed. Don't bargain with yourself or your diabetes (because it won't answer you), but make a contract with yourself and your health care providers to make things better for yourself. You can do it.

Fourth Stage: Depression

Does any of this sound familiar?

- "Why should I bother taking care of myself? I won't get my blood sugar under control anyway."
- "Being dead is better than having diabetes."
- "Now that I am a diabetic, I feel like a complete stranger to myself and to my loved ones."
- "My mother had diabetes and she lost her legs. That's what will happen to me."
- "I've never been able to lose weight, and I definitely won't be able to do it now."

"Diabetes is not the worst thing in the world. You are not alone, and you will get through this." Sure, it's easy to say this, but it's not easy to buy it. Depression is very common in people with diabetes and being told you have a chronic disease is certainly a reason to be depressed. A recent study, the DAWN Study (Diabetes Attitudes, Wishes and Needs), found that many patients find life with diabetes stressful right from the beginning, when they find out that they have diabetes.

If you find yourself depressed at any point, talk to someone. Depression can happen to anyone with diabetes. Some people do very well for several years and then reach a plateau with their diabetes care. They suddenly can't get their blood sugars lower or they stop losing weight or even start gaining weight. If a situation like this hits you, keep in mind that you have not failed. Diabetes is a progressive disease, and medications only work for so long before the body acclimates to them and they lose their effectiveness. When this happens, dosage amounts need to be adjusted or a new medication needs to be prescribed. It happens, and getting depressed about this can happen, too. If you get depressed, please talk to someone.

Words of Wisdom

You can get help directly from these experts. Dr. Rubin has written a great book called *101 Tips for Coping with Diabetes*. Bob Anderson and Marti Funnell wrote a book for diabetes educators that I personally think even patients with diabetes will love: *The Art of Empowerment*.

If depression starts to slow down your life or makes things seem impossible, then you need to talk to a doctor quickly. There are wonderful people who spend their lives helping people get through depression. There are even psychologists who specialize in caring for people with diabetes. Books and articles by Drs. Richard Rubin, Robert Anderson, Mark Peyrot, and Gary Arsham—who are leaders in the field and develop guidelines for diabetes educators in helping patients get through depression—are available and wonderful references. These people are wonderful educators and are mentors to people everywhere.

Fifth Stage: Acceptance

Does any of this sound familiar?

- "OK, so I have diabetes, but I think I can get these things under control with the help of my family and my health care providers."
- "Diabetes may be a part of me and my life from here on out, but it doesn't control my life."
- "I have diabetes; I am a person with diabetes, and I'm darn good at managing it."
- "Well, it's not going away, so I guess I really ought to learn more and take care of myself."

Hey there! You are doing much better. It really is happening, and if you take control of what's happening to you, it will be easier. Don't surrender your life to anyone. Take charge. I think you will do just fine if you decide what kind of diabetic person you will choose to be. There are two kinds of people: one who is a *diabetic* and one who just happens to *have diabetes*.

You can take control of your life and manage your diabetes or you can let diabetes control you. Which choice will you make? I like to talk about how people with diabetes are the only ones who put a sign on their heads and label

Make the Choice!

Here's a story from my first book, *Patient Education: You Can Do It!*

I met with a friend of mine, a medical director from a pharmaceutical company, and he said, "Ginger, you know I've heard you say that before, and I take exception with you."

"What do you mean?" I said.

"I am not a person with diabetes, I am a diabetic," he said. "And that's who I am. I spend more of my life taking care of my diabetes than my medical practice. I spend more of my life taking care of my diabetes and being a diabetic than being a husband or a father. I am a diabetic and I don't know if I like hearing you give me that choice."

"Well, I'm going to give you that choice," I said, "and you make the decision."

I thought about that conversation and came to this conclusion: I wish he would reconsider. Someday, when he dies—and I hope he lives to be 120 years old—what will he want said at his grave? Would he prefer people to say that he was a wonderful husband and father? A great doctor and scientist? Or a great diabetic? What do you think?

themselves *diabetics*. I try to never use that word. I have high blood pressure, and you'll never see me wearing a sign saying *hypertensive*. I don't go to a party and tell people I've just met that I'm a *hypertensive*, much like how people with cancer don't go around saying that they're *cancerous*. I am a person who happens to have high blood pressure, and I tell that to the people who need to know, such as my doctors and dentists. You are a *person with diabetes* or a *diabetic*, but which kind of person you decide to be can define how much you accept that diabetes is now a part of your life. You make the choice.

Do you see now that I will be giving you suggestions, but that I really feel that you are in charge and need to make these important decisions? Taking care of your diabetes is really your task, so the important decisions are yours to make. But I, and all of my professional colleagues, are right here to make sure you have the information you need to make the right choices for you.

TAKING CONTROL OF YOUR DIABETES

Think of your health as a ship sailing on the ocean. You need to be the captain of your ship, and this book will help you. Likewise, just as any ship needs a captain, it also needs a crew to make sure things are running smoothly. Your crew for your ship of health will be your diabetes support team. It's important to build and have a support structure. It is important that you form a partnership with your doctor and other health care providers and learn all you can about diabetes and how to deal with it. Your family and friends will also become part of your support group, if you let them, and all of you will get you through this process. When things are going well, you'll need people with whom to celebrate. Once in a while,

So, Who Is on My Crew?

Good question. Here are possible members of a diabetes support team.

- You
- Primary Care Provider (Physician)
- Certified Diabetes Educator
- Nurse Educator
- Registered Dietitian
- Eye Doctor
- Social Worker/Psychologist/Psychiatrist/Marriage and Family Therapist
- Podiatrist (foot doctor)
- Dentist
- Exercise Physiologist

I know this looks like a lot of people, but think about how many people it takes to get a space shuttle off the ground. You're basically doing the same thing but with your diabetes.

when you hit a bump in the road, they will be there for you and help you get past these obstacles.

A Crew for Your Ship

Finding the people you need to help you and forming a group to be your support structure doesn't have to be difficult. Your support group doesn't have to be formal in any way, but do decide who are the important people in your life and who you need to get through the difficult or frustrating times. Sometimes it is not your next of kin who helps you most. My husband and I get through everything together, but I wouldn't want my children making deci-

Honesty: It's the Best Policy

People sometimes lie to their doctors because they are afraid that they will be yelled at or because they don't want to disappoint the people who try so hard to make them well. I even know patients who are so fond of their health care providers that they lie to them so the educators won't feel bad that they are not doing what they were taught. Don't do this! It doesn't help anyone. I give you permission to tell me the truth. For example, if you don't eat what I suggest, then you made a choice not to. Tell me that. I'm not going to start crying or yell at you. I won't tell you that you are cheating, because how can you cheat yourself? But what we will discuss is why you chose not to eat what I suggested and what we can do to make better food choices for you. You are an adult, and I know that I and all of the diabetes educators in the world will make you partners in this process.

sions about my health care. They each have a different opinion about what is right, and they would fight about what is best for me. You need to talk to your doctor about how you want to live your life and what you are willing to do to take care of yourself. You also need to tell your care providers the truth about what you are not willing to do or not going to do. That's the key. Finding your support group doesn't need to be difficult, but it does need to be honest. You need to know and accept what your personal limits are and also acknowledge which people in your life actually help you the most.

There are wonderful people to get you to the stage where you can manage your diabetes safely and effectively. Diabetes educators are available in many communities and will work with you and your doctor to give you all of the information you need to make good decisions about your choices. They will be available for you after your classes are completed and serve as an important resource for you and your family.

Not All Crew Members Are the Same

There are still health care professionals who do not know all of the things that have happened in this fast-paced world of diabetes. So much is happening in this field that people who work in diabetes have to run just to keep current on the information. I get breathless sometimes just thinking about new insulins.

Whenever I teach a class for heath care professionals I spend the first few moments asking them questions about what they know. No one can be an expert in every aspect of the medical or health care field, so those of us who spend our lives specializing in diabetes have to bring the others along and keep them up to date. You need to make sure that the specialists you choose to fill out your crew are also knowledgeable and up to date in their diabetes skills.

If your doctor can't direct you to a diabetes educator, then you can contact the American Association of Diabetes Educators (AADE), and they will help you locate an educator in your area. You can call them at 1-800-TEAMUP-4 or visit their website at www.aadenet.org. You can also call the American Diabetes Association at 1-800-DIABETES. Either will be pleased to help you find someone to educate and help you.

If you feel your health care provider is not up on the current diabetes treatments or is not meeting your needs, you need to decide if this is the right person for you. That doesn't mean that he or she is not an excellent doctor; they may be amazing in other diseases, but they don't offer you what you need for your diabetes support team. If your ship needs new sails, you're not going to hire a carpenter to make them for you! If this happens to you, try bringing this up with your other health care partners and see who they can recommend or what they think about the situation.

Telling Others about Diabetes

Sometimes the hardest thing to do is explaining to others how you feel. It is so hard to tell someone that you are overwhelmed or that you are unsure of how to deal with something. It is easier to say nothing and keep it to yourself than to admit weakness or fear. In the middle of the night, when you can't sleep, who can you talk to about whatever is keeping you awake? Wake that person up. He or she clearly loves and cares about you if he or she is there, and I would definitely prefer if you woke them up than me. I am too far away to help.

For lots of people, it's so hard to talk about the diabetes diagnosis that it's easier to write a letter and give it to significant people in your life. After they read the letter, then you can have a discussion. Whether you have this discussion in person, face to face, over the phone, or through a letter, this conversation absolutely must happen. Make this the first step in taking charge of your ship. I know you can do it.

To make this easier for you, I've given you some sample letters that you can use to explain your diabetes and what you want these people to do to help you. You can copy these letters and fill them out or you can use these letters as an example for writing your own. Change the words to make the letter yours and write it in your own hand to make it personal. Some things never get said, but they should whenever you start a new stage in your life. These letters are to people who are important to you, so trust them with the information that you are about to give them and have faith that they will take your message to heart.

LETTER TO MY HUSBAND

Dear _____,

    I really still can't believe that I have diabetes. I keep hoping that the doctor will call and tell me that it's all a big mistake and that I have an infection that will go away with the right antibiotics. I know that it's not true, that I do have diabetes, but I'm still not happy about this whole mess. I thought this only happened to older people and overweight people. I am thin, and I exercise all the time. This really stinks.

    I know you got upset when you saw me crying the other day, but I will stop that and get on with the business of having diabetes and living well with it. I told you that I am determined to outlive you, so you can't find some young chippie and give her my jewelry.

    I want to go to that course with the diabetes educator and maybe when I understand everything, I will feel better and more in control. This is important to me; you know that I don't like anyone telling me what to do.

    Honey, please go to this class with me, so you will understand and help me get through this. I really need that. I know we have been able to get through the rough spots before. We can do anything together, right?

    Be patient when I get mad, scared, or just nasty. Hey, I may finally have that good excuse for my mood swings! I thought I would have to wait for menopause. Just think; menopause and diabetes together! You might even get sympathy from the kids.

    I just want to remind you that you love me, just as I love you.

Your name _____

LETTER TO MY WIFE

Dear _____,

   Well, it's really true. I have diabetes. I know we really don't need this at this stage of our lives, but I'm now committed to getting through this and going on with life.

   I am going to do what I can, but I am going to need your help. I am going to try my best, but I am nervous and will get nasty and annoyed. I may even snap at you at times. I was told that some people get mood swings with this condition, and it's not as if I am always easy to live with anyway. When I snap at you or other people, remind me to check my blood sugar and see if it's low. It's funny, isn't it? It will be nice to have an excuse when I blow up at the kids. "Sorry, son, my blood sugar was low."

   I will be going to see a diabetes educator and taking this course that will give me all kinds of information and tell me about eating, medications, and blood testing. I hate that idea, but the doctor says it's the most important thing I can do to manage this diabetes thing. I guess I have to buy a meter when she tells me how it works. Please go to class with me, so when I forget what they tell me, I will be able to ask you. The two of us can remember everything together.

   You will still have to shop and cook. Can you imagine me cooking anything? I will try to eat better, and I know that I have to lose some weight, but please don't nag me to death. Help and remind me, but don't get on my back all the time. I really can't stand it when you do that. If I lose some weight, I'll probably get to looking like I did when we were first married. I bet you're jealous already.

   So here we are. I better tell you now that I love you, in case I forget to later, when I really get scared.

   Your name _____

LETTER TO MY CHILDREN

Dear _____,

    Yes, it is true. I have diabetes. I am not happy about it, but it is not going to disappear, so I'm going to have to live with it and so will you. Don't be afraid for me. I will get by, and my life may be a little different, but it doesn't have to be a tragedy.

    There are things that I will have to do that might be frightening for you. I will have to test my blood with a little needle and machine. It doesn't hurt, so please don't worry. I am going to this diabetes class and will learn all kinds of things about diabetes. Your (mother/father) is going with me, and we will be in this together. If you are really worried, you can come with us and see that we're going to have everything under control.

    My dear child, I am nervous about this. It is hard to admit that I have a chronic disease and will have it for the rest of my life. I am determined to take care of myself and to do everything I can to stay well for a long time. You are free to be concerned and worry about me, but don't become a nag and a pain in the neck. I am an adult, and I will make decisions about what I will do or not do. If I ask for help with something, help me, but let me make my own decisions.

    I don't tell you enough that I love you. I do love you, and I am asking you to be part of my support group, but please remember that I am in charge of this group.

    By the way, they say when my blood sugar is low that I might get testy or nasty. What a great excuse! I love you.

(Mom/Dad)

LETTER TO MY BEST FRIEND

Dear _____,

Hi there. Guess what? I know I have been a little strange lately, but I have been worried and didn't want to talk about anything until I was sure. I have diabetes. Yeah, me. Can you believe that? I know I am a little overweight and maybe I sit around a little too much, but I didn't expect this.

I am going to get through this, and the educator told me that I need a support group. How about helping me out? You don't have to donate a kidney or anything, but I may need some help. Remind me that a light beer is OK once in a while, but I don't need all that cheese on my nachos all the time. I will learn more about what I can eat and try hard, but you might need to remind me once in a while. But please don't nag me and don't do it in front of other people.

If I get nasty at times, I mean, more than I usually am (ha ha), tell me to check my blood. I will have a meter with me; remind me that it is in my car or golf bag. By the way, how do you feel about walking the golf course instead of using the cart?

Do me a favor and don't tell everybody. Leave that to me to decide. Don't get sad or upset, either. I'll be just fine, and you will be stuck with me forever.

Thanks,
Your name _____

When discussing diabetes with your employer, it's sometimes better to wait until you're more comfortable with having the conversation. However, if having diabetes could affect your job safety or the safety of others, then you need to tell your boss right away. I don't know what you do for a living, but people with type 2 diabetes can usually do any job. However, if you require insulin, then you need to evaluate your job and your diabetes. You should discuss your particular situation with your health care provider.

LETTER TO MY BOSS

Dear _____,

    We have worked together for a long time and have a great relationship. I enjoy working for you and working here, so I want to tell you what is happening in my life. I was just diagnosed with type 2 diabetes. I am OK. I will also take really good care of myself.

    Just go on as we did before. I should not need any extra sick days and will be able to do everything that I did before. I will be testing my blood, and I don't want anyone to be scared or freak out. I don't have anything anyone can catch, so no one will get diabetes from me. I will be careful where I dispose of my needles and blood strips, so it will be safe for everyone. I will be discreet, so my co-workers and our clients don't have to know anything about it unless I choose to tell them. By the way, that decision should be up to me, so let me tell my co-workers at the right time.

    If we go out to lunch, I will know what to order, and if I choose to eat something that you don't agree with, don't say anything or nag. Please remember that I am a grown person and that I make my own decisions.

    I will continue to be a great employee and look forward to working with you for years to come. Thanks for all of your concern and consideration.

Yours truly,
Your name _____

LETTER TO MY DOCTOR

Dear Dr. _____,

   I really wanted to be angry with you and blame you for telling me that I have diabetes, but I can't. You have been telling me to watch my weight and get some exercise for years, but I thought that was just what doctors do and say to everyone, so I chose not to listen. It has taken me weeks to write this and get myself together. It has been tough getting through the past couple of weeks.

   Well, I have to accept that I have diabetes. I am angry and upset, but I will have to live with it. I will deal with this, and I want to let you know what I am going to do.

   I took your advice and signed up for a diabetes self-management education program at _____. I arranged for _____ to go with me, so I will have a partner in my care. I'll let you know how it goes.

   I will be checking my blood sugar on a regular basis and bring the results with me when I come to see you. When you go over the results, please tell me what they are telling you. I will be dealing with my weight and getting some exercise, but I really don't want you to be yelling at me or making me feel bad if I don't lose weight fast enough for you. I am an adult, and I don't want to be nagged, that doesn't work with me. Just ask my family.

   I will keep my appointments and get my blood work done when it is scheduled, as well as doing the other tests and check-ups that you advise. I am going to try, but there will be times when I just don't do what I should. That's human, right? But don't get on my back.

   I really want to take control of this, and I will. Thanks for all that you do for me, and I really know that you're concerned. I appreciate that.

   Your name _____

THE DISEASE

Have you decided to accept and take charge of your diabetes? Do you feel ready to be the captain of your ship? Have you enlisted a reliable crew to run your ship? Do the important people in your life know about your diabetes and understand what role they will play in supporting you? Great! Now that you know what to do to take charge of your diabetes, let's talk about how to manage diabetes.

Let's talk a little bit about diabetes and the different types. Remember, though, that diabetes is a chronic disease, which means it cannot be cured but can be controlled. People with diabetes are able to live long, healthy, and productive lives as long as they manage their blood sugar levels and generally take care of their diabetes.

Type 1 Diabetes

If you have type 1 diabetes, your body stops making insulin or makes only a tiny amount. When this happens, you need to take insulin to live and to be healthy. You see, without insulin, the sugar (glucose) cannot get into your cells. This is important because your cells burn glucose for energy. If glucose cannot enter your cells, then it collects in your blood. Over time, high levels of glucose in your blood may hurt your eyes, kidneys, nerves, heart, and blood vessels.

Type 1 diabetes often occurs in people under age 30. This is why it used to be called juvenile diabetes, but it can arise in anyone of any age. No one knows for sure why people get type 1 diabetes. Some people are born with genes that make them more likely to get it. But many other people with those same genes do not get diabetes. Something else inside or outside the body triggers the disease. Experts don't know what that something is yet, but they are trying to find out.

Most people with type 1 diabetes have very high levels of autoantibodies in their blood sometime before they are first diagnosed with the disease. Antibodies are proteins your body makes to destroy bacteria or viruses. Autoantibodies are antibodies that have "gone bad." They attack your body's own tissues. In these people who get type 1 diabetes, auto-antibodies may attack insulin or the cells that make insulin, which are called islet cells and are located in your pancreas.

Type 2 Diabetes

Type 2 diabetes is the kind of diabetes that is often referred to when people speak of a diabetes epidemic. If you have type 2 diabetes, your body does not make enough insulin, or has trouble using its insulin, or both. If there is not enough insulin in your body or if it's not working right, your cells cannot use the glucose in your blood to make energy. Instead, glucose stays in the blood. This can lead to high blood glucose levels, which may also lead to complications.

Most people who develop type 2 diabetes are over 40 years of age. However, a scary trend in recent years has been the increasing number of children who have been diagnosed with type 2 diabetes. Regardless of the age of a person with type 2 diabetes, many experts attribute its rising occurrence to extra calories, being overweight, and a lack of physical activity.

Experts don't know for sure what causes type 2 diabetes either. What we do know, though, is that you can't "catch" diabetes from anyone, like a cold, and that you can't develop it from eating too much sugar. Type 2 diabetes does run in families. If other members of your family have type 2 diabetes, then you are more likely to get it. Usually, though, something else has to happen to bring on the disease. A lot of research dollars are being spent to figure out what causes this switch to flip.

For many people with diabetes, being overweight brings it on. When you are overweight, your body has a harder time using the insulin that it makes. This is called **insulin resistance.** In insulin resistance, your pancreas keeps making insulin to lower blood sugar levels, but your body does not respond to the insulin as it should. After years of this, your pancreas may just burn out.

Gestational Diabetes

Gestational diabetes arises when you have high blood sugar levels during pregnancy and if you don't already have either type 1 or type 2 diabetes. It appears around 24–48 weeks of pregnancy. At that time, the body is making large amounts of hormones to help the baby grow. It is thought that these hormones block insulin from working. When something in the body does not allow insulin to do its job, **insulin resistance** develops.

In most pregnant women, the body makes enough insulin to overcome the insulin resistance. In other pregnant women, the insulin that is made cannot overcome the insulin resistance. These women have gestational diabetes. Most women with gestational diabetes have healthy babies, but there are some risks to the mother and the baby. Close follow-up by a doctor is important. Pregnant mothers are at greater risk for gestational diabetes if they

- are 25 years of age or older.
- are overweight.
- have a family history of diabetes.
- are of Hispanic, Native American, African American, Asian, or Pacific Islander ethnicity.
- have given birth to a baby weighing nine pounds or more.

Gestational diabetes usually goes away after the baby is born. But once a woman has gestational diabetes, she is more likely to develop type 2 diabetes in the future. Women who have recently given birth should have a 6-week follow-up visit with their doctor after the baby is born.

Pre-Diabetes or Glucose Intolerance

Pre-diabetes is described as having glucose levels above normal ranges but not quite at the level to diagnose diabetes. These people with pre-diabetes may not even know that they are so very close to being diagnosed with diabetes because their blood tests still fall within the normal or high-normal ranges. The American Diabetes Association is very concerned about people with pre-diabetes because there are over 41 million Americans who are walking around in jeopardy of developing diabetes. They have no idea that taking a few steps in changing their lifestyles could prevent diabetes in the near future.

Dr. David Nathan from Harvard University headed the Diabetes Prevention Program. This major, nationwide study demonstrated that type 2 diabetes could actually be prevented or delayed by catching patients with pre-diabetes and teaching them about meal planning and exercise and how to incorporate these changes into their lifestyles.

Pre-diabetes is diagnosed at different blood sugar levels, depending on the type of test used to check your blood. If you haven't eaten before having your blood sugar tested, you may have pre-diabetes if your blood sugar is between 100 and 126 mg/dl. If you undergo a more serious test, called an oral glucose tolerance test, pre-diabetes is diagnosed if your blood sugar is between 140 and 200 mg/dl.

Medications

One of the most important parts of better managing your diabetes is better managing your medications. It is such an important part of diabetes management that at each professional meeting there are days of discussion about which medications are appropriate for which patients and how medication management can be improved.

When I first started teaching diabetes education classes in the early 70s, there were three oral medications and insulin. Back then, it was difficult to get people's blood sugars under control and convincing people to go on insulin was very difficult. Diabetes management was not easy, and the prognosis for a long, healthy life was not really good. People were very frightened when faced with a diagnosis of diabetes. The options for treatment were so limited that everyone in the diabetes community was discouraged. Because of the small number of medications and their unpredictable effectiveness, diabetes educators were forced to be rigid and inflexible with their rules on what patients could and could not do. I am so glad that that era is over.

Things have changed drastically over the past 10 years. Just since 1995, over 20 new medications for the treatment of diabetes have been developed and released. There are

Getting Involved

If you would like to get involved in urging our politicians forward on important diabetes issues, go to the American Diabetes Association website (www.diabetes.org). Visit the advocacy section and see what is happening locally and nationally in regard to diabetes issues.

many more in the pipeline, but drug development takes time and an enormous amount of money. I know it can be upsetting that medications cost so much money, but the costs required to develop new medications is sometimes so high that science is caught between what needs to be done and what should be done.

Even more, medical ethics have to be considered in the development and use of medications and then the politicians get involved. You need look no further than the current debate on stem cell research and the possible cures such research may bring. But at what price? These are tough issues to consider.

WOW, THAT'S A LOT OF PILLS!

Whenever people with diabetes get together to talk about diabetes, the topic of medications always comes up. The responsibility of having to take pills or insulin for the rest of your life can be overwhelming. A patient once said to me, "I feel like a dope addict who needs his next fix." Don't fear. You're not a dope addict, and your medications shouldn't embarrass you. I bet you'd stop taking your pills right away if your doctor told you that you could. Now, what kind of dope addict does that?

If you need to take medications, then you need to take them. This is a no brainer. End of story. I know that you may hate taking pills, that it may be confusing, and that you may not be sure those medications will make a difference, but let me give you some advice about that. If you don't take your medications as directed, the consequences could be life threatening. I'm not saying this because I think that pills will "cure" your diabetes. I'm saying this because by taking your medications, you can start to get your blood sugar levels under control and help prevent those nasty complications. No one enjoys taking pills day after day after day, but you have very little choice in this matter.

I have high blood pressure. To treat this condition, I take pills twice a day without fail. Why? Because by taking these pills on time, all the time, I get to live well and be healthy. If I didn't follow this regimen, then I could have a stroke or heart attack and die. Therefore, I take my medicines. It's a pretty simple choice, right?

You have the same kinds of choices. My mother died from a heart attack when she was 55 years old, and I wasn't about to let that happen to me. The whole year that I was 55, I worried about what had happened to my mother and wondered if it would happen to me. On my 56th birthday, I called my doctor to tell him that I made it. (Now you have an idea about my age!) I am determined to live a long, healthy life, so I take care of myself, and if taking my medications will keep me alive longer and let me do the things

When the topic of medications first comes up with your doctor, you should be proactive and have a frank discussion about how you feel about taking medications and what you are willing to do to avoid them in the first place. You can say something like, "Hey Dr. Jones, I really don't like the idea of taking pills right now. I'm too young for that. Is there anything I can do right now that will keep me away from the pharmacy counter?"

I want to do, then that is the decision I choose to make. Think about your decisions.

Before You Rush Out to Buy That Pillbox

Some people hate the idea of taking pills. Others do not. If you're unafraid of medications, then you may be thinking something like this: "Give me a pill. I'll take a medicine that will take care of my diabetes, and then I can just go on living my life the way I always have. With the right pill or pills, I can continue to eat whatever I want, I won't have to exercise, and I won't get any complications or have any problems. Boy, would I like to find that miracle pill!" So would everyone else who works or lives in the diabetes community. Such a drug may be coming and things are looking very good, but it's not here yet, so you still have to make serious decisions about your lifestyle, diabetes, and medications.

When a person is diagnosed with diabetes or pre-diabetes, there is often a period of time when we look at the other ways to reduce blood sugars before going straight for the prescription pad. Why do we do this? Because over time, your body becomes more and more resistant to the drugs we give it, which means that you start taking higher and higher doses as the years pass. In order to keep you from having to take so many pills for so long and at such high costs, we try to use other methods to lower blood sugar first.

First, every newly diagnosed person with diabetes has to be given all of the information that they need to make smart, informed choices with their health care provider. Most patients are directed to start with the proven methods: blood sugar reduction, meal planning, and movement. You probably know the terms "diet" and "exercise." I hate those words. Instead, I like to call them "meal planning" and "movement." I've never seen anyone happy to be put on a diet, even though we all realize the importance of meal planning. For most people, it's even harder to motivate yourself to exercise, but we can all move. That's why instead of saying, "exercise," I say, "movement."

The next suggestion from your doctor or health care provider should be that you take a diabetes self-management education program with a diabetes education team. I know, that's a pretty long name for a class, but it simply means that the course will give you the tools and knowledge you need to take care of yourself. This comprehensive course is taught all over the country and is probably being held in your town or area right now. If your doctor or health care provider doesn't suggest this to you, then be sure to ask about it, because it's very valuable to all people with diabetes. These classes are typically outpatient programs (you only need to get a prescription from your doctor so you can be reimbursed and you need to call to reserve a spot in the class), and they are usually affiliated with a hospital or medical center. I guarantee; I will talk about this course in every chapter because I believe in it so strongly and, of course, because I am a diabetes educator.

What's Diabetes Education?

Diabetes education courses address the key issues that have been determined by the medical community to provide the best care for people with diabetes. Many of us who teach these classes add additional information that we consider important or interesting. Most courses include:

- An overview of diabetes and the diabetes process, including how it is diagnosed, the causes of diabetes, types of diabetes, and the signs and symptoms of diabetes.

Some Problems with Pills

You may love taking your medications or you may hate them, but when you have diabetes, you're going to have to take medications. There are other problems with medications, though, that go beyond simply deciding whether you like or dislike taking them. If you cannot get into a routine or you keep forgetting to take them, then that is an entirely different problem.

If you forget to take your medicine, try linking it to some other activity. I take my morning pills right after I brush my teeth and the evening ones with my first bite of dinner. If you have a favorite TV show that you watch every day, try taking your pills before that show. This will guarantee that you take your medicine the same time every day. The best way to link your medications is to think about which activities you do every day and at about the same time.

I also carry extra pills in my handbag, briefcase, and makeup kit just in case I forget to take them. Put some in your car's glove compartment or in your golf bag or fishing tackle box. Remember to refill these "stashes" before you run out, so you will always have some ready when you are forgetful. Also remember to label these pills with their names and expiration dates. Having extra supplies in handy places that go just about everywhere that you go will help you avoid being without medication wherever you are. I carry a set of my husband's pills in my handbag and I cannot tell you how many times he has had to rely on my stash. I am beginning to sound like a drug dealer. Just kidding; let's move on.

- Lessons in meal planning. This is an extensive program and may even include field trips to supermarkets to learn healthy tips. This always includes weight management and weight loss. This section is

often taught by a dietitian. It may seem like a pain,
but this part is always great fun and eye opening.

- Discussion of movement and motion. Some courses
  call this exercise, but I hate that word.
- An overview of treatment methods, including
  medications.
- Discussion of complications, including the types,
  their causes, prevention, and treatment.
- How to manage stress and risk. This session teaches
  you how to deal with living with diabetes and how
  to handle its risk factors. Some courses even include
  programs on quitting smoking.
- Tactics for changing unhealthy behaviors. This is
  often the hardest part of diabetes self-management
  education. It includes setting reasonable goals and
  problem solving.
- A description of community resources. This is so
  important because it helps you build your support
  structure and gives you access to people and organizations that can help you.
- A lesson on reimbursement and health insurance. I
  always include this because you have to pay for diabetes self-care somehow.

This is a basic course outline and most include the topics listed. Doesn't this sound like something you might like
to attend?

WHAT DO THESE DRUGS DO?

Diabetes medications do several things. They can stimulate your pancreas to make more insulin or deal with
insulin resistance. Some medications slow down the
absorption of carbohydrates. Some pills work alone, and

others must be taken with other medications. Some, like insulin, must be given by injection or inhaler. If you are put on insulin or one of the new drugs that are given by injection (pramlintide or exenatide), you need personal instruction on how to manage your injections. At the same time, don't forget that pills also have to be taken under specific circumstances, so you'll have to ask your health care provider about what rules you should follow with pills. Do you take them with food or on an empty stomach? Should you not take certain pills with other pills? These are issues that must be discussed with your doctor.

There are all kinds of new drugs coming down the road. I find this very exciting. The arsenal of weapons in the fight against diabetes is getting bigger every day. Interestingly enough, many of the new drugs being developed or released include different methods of absorption and may make a major difference in diabetes care. Soon, you might be able to take medications by wearing patches, using liquids, and administering them under your tongue. It looks like anything can happen.

DT

Your doctor may feel that your blood sugar is too high for you to wait to go on medication. If this is the case for you, then your health care provider should discuss all of the options with you. For example, your doctor might decide you need to start on a combination of drugs or even insulin right away to quickly lower your blood sugar levels. This may just need to be done for a shorter span of time. Many people believe that once you go on insulin, you can't get off it. That is just not true. Sometimes, sadly, cost is a factor as to which drugs you can take. Be sure to have a frank discussion with your health care team about which medication alternatives are best for you.

Misunderstood: Insulin

Remember, being put on insulin does not mean that you are sicker than if you just take medications or control your diabetes with diet and exercise alone. People need personalized treatments, and your doctor will determine what is best for you. If it happens that your doctor thinks insulin is best for you, then that does not mean that your diabetes is worse than that of any other person. This is often a big stumbling block in our understanding of medications. People still believe there are three kinds of people with diabetes.

1. *The Mild Diabetic:* a person who controls his or her diabetes with meal planning and motion (exercise), so his or her diabetes is not too bad or too serious.
2. *The Moderate Diabetic:* a person who takes oral medications (pills), so his or her diabetes is more serious. The Moderate Diabetic is a "real diabetic," but the situation is not dangerous and the person is not very sick.
3. *The Severe Diabetic:* a person who has to take insulin to control his or her diabetes. The Severe Diabetic is very sick, will probably get all of the terrible complications, and die young.

Do you see how wrong this is? We have always known that the best way to treat people with diabetes was to get them on the right routine and care plan for that individual. It wasn't until 1993, when the DCCT (Diabetes Control and Complications Trial) results were coming in, that we could prove that tight control really does make a difference in the prevention and treatment of diabetes complications. Since then, we are much more aggressive in the treatment of people with diabetes, and it is really making a difference in preventing the development of complications.

Remember, it is absolutely essential that you know what medications you take, their doses, and how often you take them. WRITE IT DOWN. **Put the list in your wallet and carry it with you at all times.** It is not helpful in an emergency if you tell the emergency room doctor that you take a little white pill every morning for your diabetes. You need to know the name and dose of your drugs. Your health care providers will need to know the side effects of your drugs and any possible complications that can arise from your medications. Don't depend on your doctor and health care team to always know what you take and when. You are the most important person on your health care team and should not depend on your health care professionals for everything. So please, write down your drugs.

I am going to discuss all of the medications that are available for diabetes management: what they do, their doses, and their side effects. I will tell you how they work and why they have been prescribed. I hope this will help you. I am going to describe these drugs in straightforward language, so anyone can understand it. I think this will make it clearer and easier for you because when you know what a drug does for you and how it works, it is easier to get yourself motivated to take it and understand why you should be taking it. It is also important to know that drugs may have more than one name, usually a generic name and a brand name. Knowing this will keep you from getting confused when the doctor prescribes Glucophage and your bottle comes with a label for metformin. They're the same.

Type of drug	Generic name	Brand name
Alpha-glucosidase inhibitors	acarbose miglitol	Precose Glyset

Comments: These medications stop the breakdown of carbohydrates in the intestine and prevent them from being absorbed quickly, so they slow down blood sugar increases after meals. They will not cause weight gain. They can cause low blood sugars when taken with other oral medications and can prevent the treatment of low blood sugars by preventing the absorption of carbohydrates. They often cause severe bloating and gas and need to be started with the lowest possible dose and then increased slowly. This side effect can be so uncomfortable that this medication is not used very often. It is not recommended for people with any kind of bowel problems, such as ulcerative colitis or diverticulitis.

Type of drug	Generic name	Brand name
Sulfonylurea	acetohexamide chlorpromide glimepiride glipizide glipizide (long acting) glyburide	N/A Diabinese Amaryl Glucotrol Glucotrol XL DiaBeta, Micronase, Glynase Prestab

Comments: These are the earliest oral diabetes medications, and all but chlorpromide are the newer (or second-generation) drugs. They stimulate the pancreas to make insulin and are often used in combination with other medications. They can cause low blood sugars, and the second-generation drugs are often less toxic to patients and do not affect kidney function. They are not given to patients who are pregnant and are usually the least expensive of all oral medications. Some patients are still on the earlier drugs and need to have their livers and kidneys regularly examined to make sure that they are still working properly. The sulfonylureas are mostly short-acting drugs and may need to be taken more than once daily. The XL drug is long acting and may only need to be taken once a day. These medications are not given to type 1 diabetes patients because they do not produce insulin in their pancreases, and therefore, these drugs will not stimulate insulin production.

Type of drug	Generic name	Brand name
Biguanides	metformin	Glucophage

Comments: This medication is very commonly used in people with type 2 diabetes and is often quite effective. One of the side effects is weight loss, and it often lowers cholesterol levels. This medication works on the liver and prevents it from releasing stored glucose. It rarely causes low blood sugars and, after initial side effects, usually works without problems in most people. It does have a rare side effect that must be considered, lactic acidosis, and therefore should not be given to patients with severe respiratory diseases or heart or kidney disease. Liver function tests must be done regularly.

When you are taking diagnostic tests that require radioactive iodine, such as CAT scans, you are required to notify the X-ray department that you are on metformin before the test and not take the medication the day of the exam or for two days afterwards. THIS IS VERY IMPORTANT! You may often see signs on the walls of the X-ray department reminding you to tell them about your drugs.

Type of drug	Generic name	Brand name
Meglitinides	nateglinide	Starlix
	repaglinide	Prandin

Comments: These medications stimulate the pancreas to produce more insulin for a short period of time and are taken with a meal to "cover" the carbohydrates in that meal. They are usually taken 30 minutes or less before eating a meal. Meglitinides are usually taken with other medications that cover blood sugars for the rest of the day or that may be given to deal with meals when patients are given a once-a-day injection of insulin that sets what we call a basal rate or 24-hour blood sugar goal. An example of a basal drug is Lantis insulin (also called insulin glargine). If a patient takes a meglitinide and then does not eat, then he or she could have a hypoglycemic reaction.

Type of drug	Generic name	Brand name
Thiazolidinediones	pioglitazone	Actos
	rosiglitazone	Avandia

Comments: These medications are not often given alone, but in combination with other drugs and are often the third one added to a solid oral medication attack on type 2 diabetes. They require regular liver profile blood tests before and while they are taken. They require several weeks of doses before they become effective and have been found to be quite effective in dealing with a major problem of type 2 diabetes: insulin resistance. If given to a person who takes insulin, they may allow the insulin dosage to be lowered, which may help the patient lose weight.

Type of drug	Generic name	Brand name
Combination drugs	metformin & glyburide	Glucovance
	metformin & rosiglitazone	Avandemet
	metformin & glipizide	Metaglip

Comments: You will see many drugs that are now being combined to allow you to take fewer pills and still get the medications you need. There are several combination drugs that combine sulfonylureas with biguanide or the thiazolidinediones. These drugs are usually called glitazones. Taking a combination drug allows you to get both of the medications that you require with one prescription, so it may save you money and allow you to pay one co-payment for your prescription instead of two.

INSULIN THERAPY

Insulin therapy saved the lives of countless people with diabetes. Until 1923, with the discovery of insulin, people with diabetes simply died. The discovery of insulin was the miracle of the ages, and people live long, healthy lives with insulin therapy. I have several wonderful friends who have type 1 diabetes and have received their 50-year pin from Eli Lilly, which shows that they have been taking

Please, take the time to read Dr. Gary Arsham's book, *Diabetes: A Guide to Living Well: 4th edition.* It's a great book with tons of tips about living with diabetes. Gary's also a great friend of mine, and I trust his expertise. You should, too.

insulin for 50 years and are controlling their diabetes and lives well. It is a major achievement. These people are amazing, productive, healthy, and incredible. They also happen to be diabetes educators, so they know their diabetes inside and out. I find them to be very inspiring because they show all of us how to live a life in which diabetes doesn't get in the way. They take care of themselves aggressively, test when they need to, take their insulin when they need to, and never stop working to make a difference in the lives of people with diabetes.

Insulin, Types of Insulin, and How Insulin Works

Glucose feeds, heals, and keeps the body alive and well. Glucose needs to get into the cell in order to be burned or utilized for energy. However, glucose cannot get into cells through the cell membrane without passing through a sort of door. These tiny doors into cells, called cell receptors, have to be opened by special keys. In the case of turning glucose into energy, the key to the cell just happens to be insulin. Now, can you see why insulin and glucose are so important in diabetes? If you don't have insulin to allow glucose into your cells, then you have too much glucose in your bloodstream and not enough in your cells, which causes your body to starve.

Your body does not know if you are getting insulin from your pancreas or from other, external methods. It doesn't even care. So if you are told that you need external insulin, there are several ways to get it into your body. These days, we put people on insulin much earlier in life because we know that insulin therapy is the best way to deal with diabetes, no matter whether you have type 1 or type 2 diabetes. Also, remember that insulin therapy is not simply prescribed when other medications "fail." I can't say this enough: going on insulin does not mean that you are sicker or that you have been a "bad" patient.

When I talk about "external methods" of receiving insulin, I mean the insulin that you inject either through a syringe or a pump (or now, that you inhale). But that's just the beginning. There are several different kinds of insulins that you can use for different reasons. Some act very quickly, to help your blood sugar levels during meals, and others act very slowly, to keep your blood sugar levels stable over the course of an entire day. I'll discuss these different kinds of insulins here.

Of all of the insulins, regular insulin has been available the longest, and until the development of rapid insulin, it was the most often used. Regular insulin is put in insulin pumps and is usually given intravenously (through a tube straight into your bloodstream, often called IV) in hospitals. When given in pumps or by IV, insulin starts to work immediately because it does not have to be absorbed from the injection site, such as your abdomen, arm, or leg. This means that when insulin is administered by pump or IV, it is absorbed directly into the bloodstream. Regular insulin is often combined with intermediate insulin when people with diabetes have to take two injections per day.

Analog or rapid insulin is often called immediate-acting insulin because it works almost instantaneously. It works quickly and then is gone quickly. This allows you to take your insulin just before you eat. Rapid-acting insulin eliminates the problems that arise when eating in restaurants or at any other unpredictable situation, such as at a party. Using rapid-acting insulin allows you more flexibility in planning your medications and your meals. Can you imagine taking your injection, ordering dinner in your favorite restaurant, and then your meal is delayed? You start eating the bread because you took your injection and are worried about low blood sugar, so you eat all the bread, and then your meal comes and you have a tough choice: don't eat it, take more insulin, or eat everything and have a high blood sugar reaction. If you have rapid insulin in your insulin therapy regimen, you don't have to worry about these situations as much anymore. What a relief!

Where Does Insulin Come From?

During a hot summer in 1921, two scientists in Canada, Frederick Banting and Charles Best, discovered the incredible properties of insulin use in people with diabetes. Well, actually, they first tested insulin in a diabetic dog, but then they were able to purify the insulin and bring that successful treatment to humans. Originally, insulin was made from the pancreas of a pig. That's why it was called pork insulin. Then beef insulin was developed, and both were used for many years. Beef insulin is no longer available in the U.S. because it is less reliable than human insulin.

In 1978, Eli Lilly developed Humulin, insulin that is derived from human DNA. Some patients, hearing about the new product, started calling my office to inquire about it. Many people asked me what seemed to be an obvious question: "If beef and pork insulin come from the pancreas of a cow or pig, then does human insulin come from dead people?" Of course not! All human insulins are produced synthetically in labs. If pork insulin revolutionized diabetes care, then synthetic human insulins introduced a whole new world that we never even imagined would exist.

Insulin is often taken as a combination of different types of insulins. For example, you may be taking 30 units of regular insulin in combination with 70 units of intermediate insulin. The benefit of combined insulins is that even though your diabetes may require two or even three types of insulin, you only have to take one shot instead of a different shot for each kind of insulin. Fortunately, the world has become even better! Now, you can buy premixed insulin combinations. There are several dose options, and your doctor will prescribe the one for you that will meet your needs. Insulin combinations are specific to each patient, and patients need to be trained how to properly mix their own insulins.

Some insulins, namely glargine and detemir, can't be mixed with others because they have different pH values. So, if you've been placed on combination insulin, you may still have to take more than one injection per day. It is important that you know when your insulin starts working, so you know when to eat a meal. Do you eat immediately or wait 30 minutes after you take your insulin? These are important questions.

You need to know when and how long your insulin **peaks** (meaning that it is working at its highest level of effectiveness), so you make sure you have some food in you when the medication is working at that level and don't have a low blood sugar. You should know how long it takes for the insulin to start working, which is called its time to **onset**. It is also important that you know how long the insulin will last in your body, too. This is called an insulin's **duration**. If you know this, you can plan your meals around it, remember when it will stop working, and plan to take your next dose. The more you know, the better you will be at managing your insulin. The table on page 48 will give you a good idea of how your insulin works.

	Onset	Peak	Effective duration
Rapid acting			
Insulin lispro	15–30 minutes	30 minutes to 2½ hours	3–6 hours
Insulin aspart	15 minutes	30–60 minutes	3–5 hours
Insulin glulisine	15 minutes	1–1½ hours	3–5 hours
Short acting			
Regular	30–60 minutes	2–3 hours	3–6 hours
Intermediate acting			
NPH	2–4 hours	4–10 hours	10–16 hours
Long acting			
Insulin detemir	45 minutes to 2 hours (depending on your dosage)	Relatively flat	Depends on the dose: 12–20 hours and up to 24 hours
Insulin glargine	2–4 hours	Relatively flat	20–24 hours
Inhaled insulin	15–30 minutes	30 minutes to 1½ hours	4–6 hours

Published with permission from the American Diabetes Association (*Practical Insulin, 2nd edition*).

Learn How to Take Insulin the Proper Way

Please remember that if you are put on injectable insulin, then you need to learn from a health care professional how to take your insulin. This interaction has to be face to face, as well, not through a brochure or a video. It's very hard to properly learn how to inject yourself from a book or a video. These materials are often wonderful, but they should

A Precautionary Tale

Unfortunately, good instruction in taking insulin takes a lot of time and resources, and even the best practices or facilities don't have that kind of staff, support, and time. Also, not learning the proper techniques for insulin injection can be dangerous. Let me give you an example from my own hospital and diabetes program.

One evening I was teaching a class of 12 people. We had reached the part where I let our pharmacist discuss insulin. She arrived at the administration part and was talking about the importance of rolling insulin and not shaking it before you inject it. Here's why: shaking the insulin causes bubbles that are sometimes difficult to get rid of. Bubbles in your injection can irritate your injection site and make your insulin doses unreliable, which will make your blood sugar levels unstable.

Then, one patient says, "I have been taking insulin for two years and I always shake my bottle."

I was shocked. "Well then," I asked, "how do you get the bubbles out of the bottle?"

"I don't," he replied. "I just inject them with the insulin."

I asked to see where he had given his shots and took him into an adjoining bathroom. He showed me his injection site, and I saw that his skin had a lot of bubbles under the surface. I hit the ceiling. This was unacceptable. That night, we taught him the proper way to inject himself and watched him practice until he did it correctly.

No wonder his blood sugars were so high and inconsistent! Because he injected his insulin with bubbles in the solution, his insulin doses were never the same. Those little bubbles take up room in the syringe. Now that he would be getting the right amount of insulin every time he injected, I became worried that his blood sugars would drop too quickly. So I had him call me every day for two weeks to make sure that he was safe. It's a good thing we did keep in contact because his blood sugars dropped over 100 mg/dl in a few days, and we had to adjust his insulin doses.

Stories like this are unfortunately too common, so make sure that a professional teaches you how to take your insulin until you are safe.

not replace a person who can teach you and make sure that you do it correctly.

I teach my patients how to properly inject themselves and then, to make sure that everyone has learned properly, I have them inject themselves immediately. No one leaves my class until I am satisfied that he or she is able to safely take insulin on his or her own. All of us diabetes educators want our patients to do well, and the first step in ensuring that is by making sure that our patients know how to properly take care of themselves. Do yourself a favor and make sure that you get the proper instruction that you need.

Insulin Devices

Many of the people with type 2 diabetes sincerely believe that if you are on insulin then you are seriously ill or "sicker" than other people. Therefore, they don't want to take insulin so they can avoid being labeled as a "bad" patient or as "really ill." No one wants the world to say, "You're a bad diabetic. You take insulin." But I hope that you remember what I've said earlier. These are *myths*. They are *untrue*. You take insulin to take care of your diabetes. When did it become a sign of a bad person if you're willing to do something to take care of yourself?

Another issue is that people in their 50s or 60s grew up in an era when needles and syringes were not very pleasant. They were glass and steel. They were *painful*. Many of us had inoculations or vaccinations or even antibiotic injections with these long, painful devices and that is the image we have when someone mentions injections. For many people, the mention of lifelong injections makes them panic. But there is no worry nowadays. Needle thickness is the major factor for the amount a pain you get from an injection, so the thin, disposable equipment we now have is almost pain free. I know this for a fact because I have been injecting myself with sterile saline in demonstrations for years and have felt the changes myself. Please, take my word for it. You'll be surprised.

Insulin Pens

If you still can't get over the idea of giving yourself insulin with a syringe, then maybe an insulin pen is more your speed. Insulin pens hold an insulin cartridge. When you take your insulin, you simply turn a dial and push a trigger. Insulin pens are a great invention and are very helpful for people who don't like the idea of injecting themselves or for people with arthritis or hand mobility problems. They are made by several companies and have made a major impact in the acceptance of insulin therapy among patients with diabetes.

Insulin pens are not used as commonly in the U.S. as they are abroad. They have evolved over the past few years and come in two forms: refillable pens and disposable pens that are preloaded with a certain amount of insulin. All of these devices are lightweight, nice looking, and easy to carry and use. With an insulin pen, you can easily set your dose and you never need to worry about giving yourself the wrong dose. For this reason, I recommend them for people who are visually impaired because a person who has better vision can help you set them and you won't have to worry about drawing the right amount of insulin into a syringe.

I'm afraid that one of the reasons why insulin pens are not more common is due to health insurance reimbursement. Some insurance companies will not pay for them unless there is a specific reason for the prescription, such as visual impairment. If an insulin pen sounds right for you, be sure to check your policy or options to see if pens are covered.

Insulin Pumps

Insulin pumps have been around for many years, but were not readily accepted in the beginning. Insulin pumps were complicated, and we had to very carefully select the candidates for pumps because they had to learn how to use these small, computer-like devices. Imagine what it was like for those early pump users. They had to rely on a small computer to deliver their insulin. This wasn't like programming a VCR; the stakes were much higher, and people were not as familiar with portable technology. Mistakes could cause big problems. Remember, 20 years ago, computers were not household devices.

Now this wonderful equipment is commonplace among people with type 1 diabetes and is a lifesaver for many people. The equipment is small and easy to handle. Many of the people who require insulin pumps have type 1 diabetes, so there are many children who use them. These kids have grown up with computers and other small electronics, so they think of pumps as a pretty simple piece of machinery and think that anyone who can't do this is a "doofus." Adults sometimes have more difficulty working insulin pumps than 7-year-olds, who are great at teaching their friends and family about them. I remember meeting a group of children who were all on pumps. This group travels around the country entertaining their audiences, showing how anyone can live well with diabetes and how exciting any life can be, even with type 1 diabetes. These wonderful children kept telling me how simple the pump is and that grownups make a much bigger deal out of it than they do.

Let me explain how simple insulin pumps are. A small box about the size of a cell phone holds either a syringe or cartridge filled with insulin. This insulin supply is replenished daily or every couple of days. The box is connected to a thin catheter (a small plastic tube) that is attached to a small needle. The needle is inserted into the abdomen once every three days and held to the skin by an adhesive patch. There you go. You're now hooked into a continuous, managed supply of insulin, as long as the cartridge or syringe is still filled. Now, you only get stuck once in three days instead of several times a day. The pump delivers insulin on a constant level (we call this a basal level) to keep your blood sugar at a level as close to normal as possible. Then, when you need it, you take a bolus dose of rapid-acting insulin when you eat. Pumps are now so sophisticated that you can enter your carbohydrates and they will compute how much insulin you need to give in your bolus injections for the amount of food you plan on eating.

But it gets even better. There are now insulin pumps (the Guardian RT Continuous Glucose Monitoring System by Medtronic, for example) that allow you to continuously monitor your blood sugar and give you a complete picture of how your body adapts to the foods you eat, the exercise you do, and the medications you take. These "smart" pumps also have alerts to tell you when your blood sugar is low. This is especially important for people who have hypoglycemia unawareness. People with hypoglycemia unawareness do not recognize or feel the symptoms that indicate that their blood sugar levels are dangerously low.

This is really a huge advancement in the care of children. Insulin pumps offer a wonderful blood-sugar management system and have changed the lives of many people with diabetes. Most of my colleagues who take insulin use pumps and have made them part of their lives.

Inhaled Insulin
The newest product in the insulin line is inhaled insulin and goes by the brand name Exubera. Before I go any further, I need to explain that I was hired as a consultant by Pfizer to help release Exubera to health care professionals. I have been assisting in educating diabetes educators across the country about the uses and applications of Exubera. I will give you accurate information, however, and not give you sales materials.

Inhaled insulin is a completely different way of taking rapid-acting insulin. Because it is prandial insulin (which means that it is intended to deal with glucose from the food you eat), it is taken within 10 minutes before you start to

Drug Info: Inhaled Insulin

Inhaled insulin starts to work almost immediately, like a rapid-acting insulin, but lasts as long as regular insulin (4–6 hours). It can be taken alone, in combination with oral medications, or with long-acting insulin.

It is taken by using an inhaler. The important thing to remember is that it works the same as injectable insulin and has the same benefits and complications. It is just a different way of taking your insulin. People who smoke or have lung problems cannot use inhaled insulin because the effectiveness of the insulin becomes unpredictable. I believe that lots of people who refused to take insulin before might be willing to go on insulin therapy because of this new method of taking it.

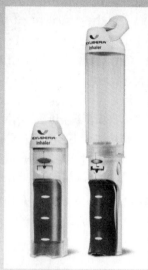

Reprinted with permission from Pfizer.

eat a meal. It is the first insulin that is given without requiring an injection, although other types of insulin are in various stages of development and may be released in the next few years.

INJECTABLE MEDICATIONS FOR DIABETES CONTROL

In 2005, two new drugs, pramlintide and exenatide, were released that have been having an amazing impact on people with diabetes. They are both injectable medications for people with diabetes.

Pramlintide (Symlin)

Pramlintide is a synthetic form of the hormone amylin, which is produced along with insulin by the beta cells in the pancreas. Amylin, insulin, and another hormone, glucagon, work in an interrelated fashion to maintain normal blood glucose levels.

Pramlintide injections are taken with meals and have been shown to modestly improve blood sugar levels without causing increased low blood sugar or weight gain. For some people, it even produces modest weight loss. No one complains about that side effect! The other side effect is nausea, which usually gets better over time and as the patient determines his or her optimal dose.

Because of differences in chemistry, pramlintide cannot be combined in the same vial or syringe with insulin and must be injected separately. Pramlintide has been approved for people with type 1 diabetes who are not reaching their blood sugar goals and for people with type 2 diabetes who are using insulin and are not reaching their blood sugar goals.

Exenatide (Byetta)

Exenatide is the first in a new class of drugs for the treatment of type 2 diabetes called incretin mimetics. Exenatide is a synthetic version of exendin-4, a naturally occurring hormone that was first isolated from the saliva of the lizard known as a Gila monster. It lowers blood glucose levels primarily by increasing insulin secretion. Because it only has this effect when there are higher blood sugar levels, it does not tend to increase the risk of blood sugar lows. Be aware, though, that blood sugar lows can occur if exenatide is taken with a sulfonylurea. The primary side effect is nausea, which also tends to go away over time.

Like pramlintide, exenatide is injected with meals and patients using it have generally lost a little weight and improved their blood sugar levels. Exenatide has been approved for use in people with type 2 diabetes who have not achieved target blood sugar levels using metformin or a combination of metformin and a sulfonylurea.

GLUCAGON INJECTIONS

Glucagon is a hormone produced in the pancreas. It raises blood sugar levels and is given for severe hypoglycemia reactions. If your blood sugar has gotten so low that you cannot eat food or drink liquids to raise your blood sugar, this becomes a life-threatening emergency and requires an injection of glucagon. You can purchase a **glucagon emergency kit**, so you can be prepared for just such an emergency. A glucagon emergency kit contains one dose of glucagon in powder form and a sterile liquid that must be mixed with the glucagon powder. This solution is then given as a direct injection into the muscle and has an immediate effect. Generally, glucagon is needed and used only by people with type 1 diabetes. Discuss with your health care provider whether you should carry this medication, but I certainly think that every person with diabetes should have glucagon ready in case of an emergency.

You should also carry glucose gel or glucose tablets with you and have them available in your car or workplace. This is not meant to scare you, but to prepare you for events that do occur when you have diabetes.

ADDITIONAL MEDICATIONS

Many people with diabetes take additional medications to deal with other problems. We call these other problems that often accompany diabetes **comorbidities**. The list of comorbidities for diabetes goes on and on and so does the list of medications for them. There are medications that tackle elevated cholesterol and triglyceride levels, high blood pressure, and all of the other complications of diabetes.

All people with diabetes should have a flu shot every year and a pneumonia vaccination every 10 years. Remember, prevention is always better than having to deal with a problem once it occurs. Be proactive!

Not only are various ways of taking your medication available, but you may need to take drugs for any number of conditions. Some people may require medications to deal with their blood pressure or cholesterol levels. You should pay attention to your lipid levels (cholesterol and triglyceride), so you may need medications for

An Example of Over-the-Counter Problems

Some people take a supplement called chromium picolinate because they believe that it may reduce blood sugar levels. It is sold over the counter, too. But if you take this supplement, you need to consider what might occur if you take it with other medications that lower your blood sugar. If both do work, then you may be risking constant low blood sugar levels, which can be dangerous. If you do take over-the-counter supplements like chromium picolinate or anything else, please tell your health care providers. They will be able to bring their knowledge and experience to your aid and show you what medications and medication combinations will work best for you.

The American Heart Association and the American Diabetes Association recommend that, when possible, people who have diabetes and are 45 years old or older should take one children's aspirin a day. A children's aspirin has a dosage of 81 mg, so look for this amount when you're at the local drug store or supermarket. But don't grab your car keys just yet. For some people, taking aspirin daily may counteract some of their prescribed drugs or affect a current health condition, so meet with your doctor before starting aspirin therapy. See how this works? Always talk to your health care providers before taking any new medications or supplements.

that as well. I know, by now, I'm driving you crazy. It probably sounds like I am just going through the pharmacy and naming all of the drugs! I'm not, even though it may sound like it. In many cases, people with diabetes need to take a lot of medications.

I ask all of my patients to bring a list of all of their medications to me, and I don't just mean the prescriptions. It can also be very dangerous to combine prescription drugs and over-the-counter medications, such as allergy pills and decongestants. If you buy nutritional supplements, such as St. John's wort or Echinacea, in health food stores or over the Internet, or from wherever, they need to be brought to the attention of your health care providers. Let me explain. Many medications were originally developed from plant extracts or are made from natural foods. If you take one prescription drug that has belladonna in it and then take a supplement in it with belladonna, then you are getting two doses of belladonna. When medications are concerned, there is such a thing as too much of a good thing.

CONCLUSION

There are thousands of different medications, and you may be required to take one or several of them during your diabetes lifetime. So many people are willing to take a pill because their doctor told them to and don't investigate the alternatives, what the pill is supposed to do, and what are the dangers involved with taking it. Don't let this happen to you. Ask questions. We all have a responsibility to know our options in health care and take responsibility for the drugs we take.

This is understandable, though. Often people are afraid to ask their doctors too many questions. They don't want to seem stupid, naïve, or ignorant. Don't sweat it. Even the most educated person in the world cannot know everything about anything, and a phrase has been developed to make us all understand this better: **health care literacy.** This term describes how knowledgeable you are about health care in general. No one is completely literate in health care. You cannot know all the jargon and phrases in medicine. So, please feel free to ask. When you pick up your prescription, you have a great partner, your pharmacist. A major part of his or her job is patient education—improving your health care literacy. Sometimes, people forget that part.

Have you ever picked up your prescription and been asked to sign a paper with little white labels added to it? Most people think that sheet tells your insurance to pay for the drug. If you look at the top of the paper, you'll see that you are signing a form that states that you don't need any information or education about the medication. Did you know that? Don't sign away your right to information and education or to health care literacy. Make sure you take the time to ask questions. With proper health care literacy and education, you can take your medications safely and improve your life overall. Safety is not a joke, so don't feel embarrassed when you want to know about those little pills.

Three

Meal Planning

et's talk about everyone's favorite subject, food. Unless you have diabetes, that is. When diabetes is involved, eating suddenly turns into a complicated activity. Meal planning becomes a major part of your life, and you cannot just go your merry way and eat everything in sight. So let's take a long look at what you are eating and what you should be eating.

Food is everywhere—on TV shows, billboards, and magazines, and it's even splashed across the Internet. We talk about what we ate last night, what we will eat today, and what we will eat for dinner tomorrow. So much human activity seems to involve food. And why not? Eating keeps us all alive. You cannot avoid eating food, and it seems almost cruel when you have to watch what you eat to stay healthy or lose a few pounds. If you have diabetes, though, you'll have to start eating healthily and that means that you'll have to create a **meal plan.**

You'll notice that I did not say anything about a **diet.** That is such a terrible word. When I talk to large groups of people about their diabetes, I always ask how many of them have ever been on a diet. Most of them will always raise their hands. I then ask how many of them couldn't follow that diet, and they all raise their hands. This chapter isn't about diets, it's about meal planning. There is a difference.

DIABETIC DIETS: FACT OR FICTION?

An elderly lady in a nursing home once said to me, "I weigh 85 pounds, and they have me on some stupid diet. Can you imagine?" You may feel the same way when you meet with your doctors and other health care providers.

To most people in the world, the word **diet** means eating less to lose weight. Although many people with diabetes should lose weight, a meal plan is primarily designed to help you manage your blood sugar levels. Weight issues are generally, but not always, a secondary goal. As someone with diabetes, you will have to follow a meal plan.

Before we get too far into this, though, you need to forget all that stuff you've heard about **diabetic diets**. Give up on the idea that your doctor is going to hand you a piece of paper that will show you how to eat for the rest of your life. First of all, that would get pretty boring really fast. Can you imagine eating the same meals day after day after day? Moreover, because the task of caring for your diabetes is so complicated, these so-called diabetic diets don't really exist.

Keyword: Diabetic Diet

If you have diabetes, then you've heard this term before. A diabetic diet is supposed to be the diet that people with diabetes should follow. It gives you specific and clear rules on what to eat and what to avoid so you can keep your blood sugars under control. Foods are divided into "good" and "bad" types. Lots of people with different conditions have diets tailored to their conditions; for example, people with celiac disease have to follow a gluten-free diet. Unfortunately, things aren't that clear cut when you have diabetes.

Sure, people with diabetes have been given diabetic diets before and lots of people out there will try to sell you on a diabetic diet, but they have not been used for over 10 years. You see; these so-called diabetic diets offer only a very simple, sometimes unhealthy approach to taking care of your diabetes. There are no "good" or "bad" foods when you try to eat healthily with diabetes; it just matters how much and how often you eat these foods. Now, you may occasionally see a printed version of a 1,800-calorie diabetic diet from the American Diabetes Association. Here's why. Years ago, the American Diabetes Association and the American Dietetic Association developed and issued some diet guidelines, but since then, we've learned a lot about diabetes and realized that a strict diabetic diet is counterproductive. Nevertheless, these old diets are still in existence and are still being used in some areas.

Some health care professionals, who do not spend their entire lives dealing with diabetes, may not have enough time or experience to do a major session on meal planning with you and may give you a "diabetic diet." These diets may offer a good place to start so you can get important information about meal planning, start thinking about eating healthy food, and work yourself into the mindset that you have to watch what you eat. At this point, I really hope that you are referred to a registered dietitian, who may or may not be a certified diabetes educator. If not, bring this up with your doctor. A registered dietitian will have the time and experience to help you with your meal plan far more than some sheet with a "diabetic diet" on it. These rigid diets can still be helpful, but an individualized meal plan works much better. If a person with diabetes hasn't eaten well for decades, it's going to take some work getting him or her to think healthy and these older diets may provide a great starting point.

So what can you do to get started and who can help you? Ask your health care provider if he or she has some materials on meal planning for diabetes or a diabetic diet. Just because we discuss meals plans doesn't make the other ones forbidden or completely wrong. Start looking at these materials and compare what they suggest to what you have already been eating. That's a great place to start. Maybe you're lucky, and you won't have to make many changes at all.

Do You Cheat?

I always hear people talking about cheating on their diets. It often shows up as a question. "Have you been cheating on your diet?" A family member will sometimes say, "Oh, he cheats on his diet." I have a question in response to that. Who is cheating here? What has he or she cheated on? It's a strange expression. You can't cheat on a diet. When you don't follow a diet, you make a decision and you have to take responsibility for making that decision. The more important question is why you decided not to follow the diet. So let's stop calling it cheating.

LET'S MAKE A MEAL PLAN

Remember, you have been eating the same way for your entire life, and now you're being told that you need to change some things to stay healthy. These are big changes because they affect your lifestyle, the way you live your life. There is no way you will be able to change everything immediately, and no one expects that of you. You will need to make reasonable changes that you can achieve, so shooting for the stars will not help. So don't go out there and tell me that your new healthy goal is to lose 50 pounds in two months. I don't believe you when you say that, and I'm pretty sure you don't believe yourself either.

Because you've been eating this way for years, what you like to eat, when you eat, and how you eat have become habits, which is why we call them **eating habits.** Everyone has eating habits, so don't think you're the only one with them. Eating habits are hard to break, which is why so many of those quick-fix diets don't work. Quick-fix and short-term diets never address changing your eating habits over the long term, so once you've finished the diet's time-line, you go back to your old ways of eating. But not all eating habits are bad. Most do lead to weight gain or loss, though, and altering unhealthy eating habits is one of the primary goals of meal planning.

I know, by now you're probably thinking, "Ginger, this doesn't sound easy at all! Just give me that diabetic diet. Meal planning sounds like arranging a wedding, and that's one serious pain in the rear!" I understand where you're coming from, but meal planning doesn't have to be difficult or painful. In fact, the rationale behind it is really quite simple. Will changing your lifestyle to follow a meal plan be difficult? Yes, it will. But I don't think you'll find it to be as hard as you imagine. I highly recommend that you make an appointment with a **registered dietitian.** Many patients

Some Sample Eating Habits

- Eating in front of the TV
- Dessert is a must-have course in any meal
- I eat salad for the salad dressing; those vegetables are for the birds
- Skipping breakfast
- Eating in the car
- Standing up while eating
- Finishing everything on your plate all the time
- Eating as much as you can at a buffet

Keyword: Registered Dietitian

A registered dietitian is a health care professional who advises people about meal planning, weight control, and diabetes management. This person will be a very valuable asset to your health care team, so try to meet with one as soon as possible. I bet it's getting tiring listening to me say this again and again, but that's because having a dietitian help you is so very, very important. You can find a registered dietitian by calling the American Dietetic Association at 1-800-877-1600 or by going to www.eatright.org.

are covered by their health insurance plans for three hours of medical nutrition therapy during the first year after diagnosis and then for two hours every year after that. These hours are in addition to the materials on meal planning taught in a complete diabetes education program. Setting up that appointment may be the best thing you ever do.

THE BASICS OF MEAL PLANNING

A dietitian's job is to talk to you about what you eat now and how to make adjustments to ensure that your body is not badly affected by the foods you eat. When I am teaching a diabetes class, I spend hours and hours on meal planning. Because you're reading this book, you won't be able to ask me questions, but I'll try to give you as much information as possible. And, of course, I'm going to refer you to a dietitian again, because he or she will make all of this a lot clearer than I can in one chapter.

The first step is to look at what and how much you're already eating. People with diabetes often think that if they skip a meal, then it will be better for them. I can understand why *all* people make this mistake: if you take in fewer calories by skipping a meal, then you're going to lose some weight. But here's something strange. It seems to me that the people I know who skip meals (and especially breakfast) are always the people who are overweight. So, I've got some bad news for you: skipping meals will not solve your problems. Here's what really happens when you skip a

Recommendations for a Healthy Meal Plan

The National Diabetes Education Program—a partnership of the National Institutes of Health, the Centers for Disease Control and Prevention, and more than 200 public and private organizations—suggests these tips in creating a healthy meal plan.

- Eat a variety of foods as recommended in the Food Pyramid to get a balanced intake of the nutrients your body needs: carbohydrates, proteins, fats, vitamins, and minerals.
- Make changes gradually because it takes time to accomplish goals that last.
- Reduce the amount of fat you eat by choosing fewer high-fat foods and cooking with less fat.
- Eat more whole grains. Most people think that the only whole grain is whole wheat. Oats, corn, and bulgur are also whole grains. They provide you with more vitamins, minerals, and fiber than refined grains.
- Eat more fiber.
- Eat fewer foods that are high in sugar, such as fruit juices, fruit-flavored drinks, sodas, tea, or coffee sweetened with sugar.
- Use less salt in cooking and at the table. Eat fewer foods that are high in salt, such as canned and packaged soups, pickles, and processed meats.
- Eat smaller portions and never skip meals.
- Learn about the right serving sizes for you.
- Learn how to read food labels.
- Limit your use of alcohol.

meal, especially breakfast. You get up in the morning and skip breakfast, and by the time lunch comes around, you are so hungry that you eat everything in sight. The best way not to be hungry is to eat small, frequent meals, so you never feel starved or deprived. That way, you are not walking around waiting for your next meal.

This small, frequent, meal plan idea makes even more sense if you think about how diabetes affects your body. In people with diabetes, either your body is not making enough insulin to deal with the meals you eat or it is resistant to your own insulin. Regardless, your pancreas becomes stressed from the demand for insulin and cannot keep up. Now, if you ate smaller meals more frequently, you would not be stressing your pancreas quite so much because there would be less demand for large amounts of insulin to cope with large meals. That is why I recommend that you eat six small meals a day: breakfast, lunch, dinner, a mid-morning snack, an afternoon snack, and a pre-bedtime snack.

Using the Food Pyramid

A great way to get involved in choosing healthy foods is by using the food pyramid. Now, I'll bet that you're unfamiliar

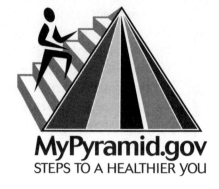

From left to right, the bars represent the following food groups: grains, vegetables, fruits, oils, milk, and meats and beans. The exact daily amounts rely on your age, gender, weight, and activity level, which you can find out by visiting www.mypyramid.gov.

MyPyramid.gov
STEPS TO A HEALTHIER YOU

with the one in this book. This food pyramid has been revised by the U.S. Department of Agriculture. You will notice immediately that exercise has been added to the staircase and it shows how important diet and exercise are in combination. This pyramid shows you all of the foods that go into planning daily meals and how much each kind of food should fit into your meals every day. The sections are different sizes, which is helpful in showing that you should, for example, eat less fats than vegetables. It will help you think about the portions of food you choose, too. Go to www.mypyramid.gov and play with all the sections

A Word about Calories

Let's talk about calories for a moment. We all look at the calories in a food when we buy it, but there's more to that little number than just calories. Each type of food—carbohydrates, protein, and fat—has its own calorie value. Carbohydrates and protein each carry a value of 4 calories per gram. Fat has 9 calories. Now do you see why eating a small fatty food adds more to your waist than a bigger, less fatty food? For example, if a food label says that the food has 10 grams of fat, then that means it has 90 calories from fat (10 × 9 = 90 calories). So think carefully when you look at two bags of potato chips and one has 5 grams of fat and the other has 11 grams of fat.

A lot of people count calories, and it is a valid way to measure how much you are eating. More and more people with diabetes are looking at the amount of carbohydrates they eat because "carbs," as we call them, are what raise your blood sugar the most. There is a problem with just looking at carbs, though. When we eat low-carb foods, we may not look at all the fat calories in them. Those fat calories will add to your weight, probably your waist. So keep an eye on those calories, always.

on the site to get a personalized pyramid made just for your needs.

Food Diaries

You will be asked to keep a record of what you eat for the next three days, which is what we call a **food diary**. This can be tough, and it is a real chore to write down everything you eat every day, but you can do it. Most important, remember to be truthful because no one is going to yell at you or think you are stupid when they read it. Your health care providers are going to analyze it to see what you do well and what can be done better. In fact, the toughest part will require you to be honest with yourself. When you actually write it down and see it, you will be amazed at the amount and kinds of foods that you eat in a single day. After you complete this food diary, bring it to your diabetes educator or dietitian and start the process of becoming a healthy eater.

Time	Food	Food preparation	Amount you eat

From *Diabetes Meal Planning Made Easy, 3rd Edition*, by Hope S. Warshaw.

Here are some things to keep in mind while you fill out your food diary:

- write down everything you eat
- enter what time you ate it
- describe what the food was
- describe how much of the food you ate

Here's another thing: you need to consider the components of the foods you eat. So, for example, when you eat a cheese sandwich, you should write down that the sandwich had tomatoes, mayonnaise, roast peppers, cheddar cheese, and two slices of bread. All of these little ingredients need to be counted by your dietitian.

When discussing a food diary, you and your health care provider will look for lots of things, such as how often you eat, what times you eat, what kinds of foods are your favorites, and what foods you tend to avoid. We also look at the amounts of food you eat or the portion sizes. One of my patients will not eat a salad, no way, no how. He simply refuses to eat that "grass junk." This makes for a challenge, but we have been able to work around it. You see, keeping a food diary allows us to create a meal plan approach that works *for you*.

It is important to watch what you eat, but in a lot of ways, what we look for when we review a food diary is your food portions. Moderation is the name of the game when it comes to taking care of your diabetes. We used to measure everything with measuring cups or measuring spoons, but many dietitians now recommend using small food scales, so your measurements are precise. A lot of this new emphasis on scales has come along because we have all relied on sloppier methods of measuring portions in the past. If you use a measuring cup or spoon, after a while you begin to "see" the measurement. Over time, this becomes less and less precise, which will affect your overall health. Can you remember the

The only way to truly tell portion size on a consistent basis is to weigh the food you are going to eat. That means you should get a food scale. This doesn't mean that you have to lug this piece of equipment around with you every time you eat out, but when you cook at home, use it. Food scales can be ordered from the Internet or found in kitchen supply stores, such as Williams-Sonoma or Sur La Table. They are not hard to find and will make your life much simpler. Try to get the most accurate one you can afford.

last time you tried to measure something's size with just your hands? How precise were those measurements when you compared them to an actual ruler or measuring tape? The same applies to food measurements. If you just rely on measuring cups and spoons and your "eye," then you'll occasionally have to "recalibrate" your skills.

Here's how a friend of mine "recalibrates" herself. She's a diabetes educator and has had type 1 diabetes for over 40 years, so she's not just doing this for fun. Once every 6 months, she takes out her measuring cups and spoons and pours portions of food onto plates and bowls to remind her of what a cup or a tablespoon of food really looks like.

KNOW YOUR NUTRIENTS

Food is divided into **carbohydrates, protein,** and **fat,** but the one we are most concerned with is carbohydrate. Carbohydrates are particularly important in people with diabetes because they are converted to glucose that enters your bloodstream and raises blood sugar levels. Remember,

Keyword: Blood Fats

Keeping your blood fats down is every bit as important as lowering your blood sugar. People with diabetes have a much higher rate of heart disease than anyone else, so this is critical. You've probably heard of lipids and cholesterol before. Well, lipids are fats stored in the body, and cholesterol is fat found in the bloodstream. Hardened and clogged arteries are the results of high levels of certain types of cholesterol. When you hear that someone has had a triple or quadruple heart bypass surgery, this is often due to having high cholesterol levels over a long period of time. These are important issues, and people with diabetes must also pay attention to the foods they eat so they can lower their risk of having high cholesterol levels.

glucose needs to get into the cells in order to be used for energy. So when people tell you to watch your sweets because you have diabetes, this is not exactly right. Many sweets do contain a lot of carbohydrates, but so do many other foods, so if you have diabetes, you'll need to watch for all foods that contain carbohydrate. Bread, potatoes, grains, milk, yogurt, fruits, and vegetables are just some of the carbohydrates that people never consider.

Carbohydrates

There are three primary kinds of carbohydrates: **starches, sugars,** and **fiber.** On the nutrition label on foods, the term "total carbohydrate" includes all three types of carbohydrates. This is the number you should pay attention to if you are carbohydrate counting (but I'll have more on this later, see page 81). Still, it's not going to hurt you if you know more about carbohydrates, so I'm going to give you a quick lesson in nutrition.

Starches

Starches are composed of many long chains of glucose that are hooked together, which is why they are sometimes called **complex carbohydrates.** You've probably heard this before, a long time ago in school, and forgotten it since. I know a lot of people who have. But you're not here for a lecture on chemistry and the structure of molecules, so I'll just give you the details you need.

Sugars

Sugars, in contrast to starches, are composed of single chains of glucose, fructose, or lactose, which is why they are sometimes called **simple sugars.** Because they are just single chains of a sugar, though, doesn't mean that they affect your blood sugar levels any faster or more dramatically than the glucose derived from starches. Fructose is a sugar that is found in fruit, and lactose is a sugar found in milk. Are those old chemistry lectures coming back to you now? Me neither.

Sugars include honey, molasses, syrups (such as corn syrup and maple syrup), processed sugars (such as table sugar, brown sugar, and powdered sugar), and natural sug-

---

Foods That Are High in Starch

- Starchy vegetables, such as peas, corn, lima beans, and potatoes
- Dried beans, lentils, and peas, such as pinto beans, kidney beans, black-eyed peas, and split peas
- Grains, such as oats, barley, and rice (bread and pasta are included in this category)

A Spoonful of Sugar

There's another type of sugar that people often see, table sugar. Table sugar is also called by its chemical name, sucrose. Do you see a trend yet? When you see the chemical name for a sugar, it ends in "-ose," like in sucrose, glucose, and lactose. There are other sugars, such as maltose, and some surprises, too. Did you know that dextrose is another name for glucose or that fructose is also called levulose? Now, whenever you're looking at a food label, you'll be able to see that the ingredients contain added sugar if you see any of those -ose words.

I have a hunch that over the years, a lot of people with diabetes have been told to avoid desserts because people are confused about the different types of sugar present in food. Mention sugar and a lot of people just think of table sugar (sucrose), sugar cookies, and sugary cake frosting. As you can see, that's not exactly the same kind of sugar as when you're talking about your blood sugar. People rarely think about the sugar (or, more specifically, glucose) that you get from pasta, breads, peas, some beans, and other carbohydrates when diabetes comes up in conversation.

So I'm going to do some myth busting for you because I go through the roof whenever a person tells me that eating sugar gives you diabetes or that people with diabetes can't ever enjoy a cookie. *You can eat foods that contain sugar.* But (you knew a "but" was coming, didn't you?), you have to work them into your meal plan, just like you would any other food that contains carbohydrates. As with everything else you eat, you're going to have to eat foods that contain sugar in moderation and with an eye toward how they affect your blood sugar levels.

ars (such as lactose in milk and fructose in fruits). Foods with natural sugars are usually good sources of nutrients, such as vitamins, minerals, fiber, and protein. Many other nutritious foods, such as breakfast cereals, breads, and low-fat salad dressings, contain some added sugars. Some other foods with added sugar, such as chocolate, baked treats, and ice cream treats, provide lots of calories and fat, with few nutrients in return. When it comes to foods with added sugar, you'll generally have to be selective when choosing them for your meal plan.

Fiber

Fiber is the part of plant foods, including fruits, vegetables, whole grains, nuts, and legumes, that your body cannot digest. When you eat fiber, most of it just passes through your digestive system. Fiber is good for you. Fiber keeps your digestive system healthy, keeps your bowel movements regular, and helps you feel full and satisfied after a meal. No one these days seems to get enough fiber. In fact, most Americans only get about one-half of the amount of fiber we should be getting each day. The average adult should be eating about 25–30 grams of fiber each day and so should you. Try to get your fiber from foods and not supplements because, in addition to being a great source of fiber, fiber-rich foods normally have a wealth of other important vitamins and minerals.

Good sources of dietary fiber include the following:

- Fruits and vegetables, especially those with edible skin (such as apples, corn, and beans) and those with edible seeds (such as berries).
- Whole grains, such as whole-wheat pasta, whole-grain cereals, and whole-grain breads.

- Beans and legumes, such as black beans, kidney beans, pinto beans, chickpeas, white beans, and lentils.
- Nuts, such as peanuts, walnuts, and almonds, but be careful with them, because nuts also pack in a lot of calories in a small package.

Carbohydrates and Meal Planning

Take a look at this list of carbohydrate foods:

- Breads
- Cereals
- Crackers and snack chips
- Grains
- Pasta
- Dried beans, peas, and lentils
- Vegetables
- Fruits
- Sweets
- Sugary foods
- Milk and yogurt

Think about this list for a moment. Are these foods good or bad? Which ones? Why? As with all things related to diabetes, the answer isn't so easy. There is no such thing as good or bad foods, there is only food, and some are better for you than others. There are no foods that you can never eat—there are foods you should avoid or eat less of, though—but you need to make choices and eat in moderation.

Remember, an important task in meal planning, especially when you do have diabetes, is being able to identify which foods contain carbohydrate and will therefore most influence your blood sugar levels. It does not really matter where you get your carbohydrates, but you do need to know what foods are carbohydrates and how many grams of them you eat per day and for each meal and, if needed, each snack. You will need to meet with a dietitian in order to determine how many carbohydrates are best for you and in what proportion per meal. Most of this depends on your weight, lifestyle, medications, and BMI (body mass index, which is a measurement that accounts for your weight in relationship to your height). A healthy BMI falls into the range of 19–24.9 kg/m². I also know that there's been a lot of talk about how normally fit people are categorized as overweight due to their BMI number. This is because BMI only offers a generalized picture of a person's body mass, so athletes, for example, tend to weigh more than people of the same height because they have more muscle mass. This is just another reason why you'll be better aided by meeting with a dietitian, who can meet with you and help you develop a personalized meal plan.

So, just to give you an idea of what meal planning really takes, I've got a fun activity for you. Here is a list of foods. Circle the foods that contain carbohydrates.

Locate the Carbohydrate Foods

- Old-fashioned oats
- Barley
- Spinach
- Cottage cheese
- Pork chop
- Banana
- Bran flakes
- Broccoli
- Sugar-free cookies
- Catsup
- Balsamic vinegar
- Green tea
- Tuna
- Low-fat salad dressing
- Lentil soup
- Chicken cutlets
- Whole-wheat bread
- Low-carbohydrate pasta

Developed by Lorena Drago, RD, MSN, CDE

Are you ready for the answers? You may be surprised by some. All of the bold foods contain carbohydrates.

- **Old-fashioned oats**
- **Barley**
- **Spinach**
- **Cottage cheese**
- Pork chop
- **Banana**
- **Bran flakes**
- **Broccoli**
- **Sugar-free cookies**

- **Catsup**
- **Balsamic vinegar**
- Green tea
- Tuna
- **Low-fat salad dressing**
- **Lentil soup**
- Chicken cutlets
- **Whole-wheat bread**
- **Low-carbohydrate pasta**

I know. It probably looks overwhelming trying to remember which foods fall into each category. There are some helpful tools out there to make your job easier. First off, start reading food labels. They tell you exactly what category that particular food will fit in. For instance, if you pick up a package of frozen strawberries, you'll see that the label shows how many carbohydrates are in it. The label will also show you the portion size and tell you how many calories are in the portion. Frozen fruit are great because fresh fruit and vegetables do not have food labels but packaged frozen foods do. Does this mean that you should only eat frozen fruits and vegetables? No way! But you can learn from the food labels on frozen foods and start to see what you'd get from fresh fruits and vegetables. The food exchange lists from the American Diabetes Association are also great tools. These booklets divide foods into their proper categories and show you how to fit them into your meal plan.

Quick Reference Guide to Carbs

Here's a brief, easy way to think about how to fit carbohydrates into your daily meal plan.

Choose Often
- Bean, peas, lentils
- Fresh fruits
- Vegetables
- Skim or 1% milk/yogurt
- Whole grains: oats, oat bran, 100% whole wheat, rye, pumpernickel, barley, brown rice

Choose Occasionally
- Breads, bagels, muffins, crackers made with white flour
- Enriched wheat flour
- White rice
- Fruit juice and drinks
- Whole milk or 2%
- Regular sodas/drinks

When you start making choices about healthy eating, there are no forbidden foods, but some foods might be better for you until you get a grip on setting up your own meal plan.

Further Reading

I'm also going to refer you to two amazing dietitians and their wonderful book. This resource will take you through all of the information and give you clear and concise instructions on how to get those carbohydrates under control and counted. You will not find better educators anywhere, and this book won't let you down. This book is the *Complete Guide to Carb Counting* by Hope S. Warshaw and Karmeen Kulkarni.

Carbohydrate Counting

Now that you know which foods contain carbohydrates and how to identify them, let's talk about a vital tool in meal planning for people with diabetes: carbohydrate counting.

Now, whenever you eat any meal or snack, it is usually a mixture of carbohydrate, protein, and fat. As I have pointed out, the carbohydrate is converted to glucose, which powers your cells and also can lead to high blood sugar levels if you have diabetes. In carbohydrate counting, you count foods that are mostly carbohydrate. These include starches, fruits and fruit juices, milk, yogurt, ice cream, and sugars. You do not count most meats

or fats. These foods have very little carbohydrate in them.

You can find out how much carbohydrate a food has by looking at the *Exchange Lists for Meal Planning: Basic Carbohydrate Counting,* the food label on food packaging, or by asking your dietitian.

Knowing how much carbohydrate a food has can help you better manage your blood sugar levels. If you take at least three or four doses of insulin a day or use an insulin pump, you will have to learn to adjust each insulin dose to cover the amount of carbohydrate you eat. If you do not take insulin, you can learn how to space carbohydrate throughout the day to improve your blood sugar levels.

Protein

Proteins are foods that mostly come from living things: meat, fish, eggs, milk, cheese, and milk products. Certain vegetables and other things that grow, such as beans, also contain protein. Here's a pretty easy way to instantly know which foods contain protein. My friend, Lorena Drago, teaches her patients that most protein foods used to have a face. Think about all of the animals that have a face. Cows, pigs, chickens, fish, and turkeys all have faces, so beef, pork, chicken, fish, and turkey are all protein foods. So, if that animal got off the ark with Noah, then you're eating protein.

I can hear you saying it already: "Ginger, protein doesn't really raise blood sugar levels, so I'm going to eat more protein and fewer carbohydrates. I really like that idea." Well, that's not the best idea in the world. Lots of protein foods come from animals, so they are usually loaded with animal fats as well, which can add more saturated fat and cholesterol to your diet. This is not what a person with diabetes wants to add to his or her meal plan. Don't forget, protein foods also have a lot of calories. Too many unspent calories usually result in weight gain, which will make it even harder for you to manage your diabetes.

When eating, go for the healthier bets, of which I'm pretty sure you're already aware. You know, get your chicken without the skin, order leaner cuts of meat, go with fish and seafood instead of land-based animals for your meats, and choose low-fat or nonfat milk, cheese, cottage cheese, and other dairy products. Great sources of protein without a face include legumes (beans, peas, and lentils), grains, and vegetables because they are low in fat, have fewer calories, and have no cholesterol. Nuts and seeds are also great options. They have lots of protein, and the fat they contain is usually unsaturated.

Dietary intake guidelines suggest limiting your protein intake to 10–35% of your total calorie intake. You need protein in your diet to build tissues and muscles, and it contains many nutrients that you need to maintain a healthy body. The problem is that most Americans eat much more protein than they need. Even more, many restaurants promote and sell much larger steaks and burgers than most humans should ever consume. Does your body really need a 20-ounce steak?

It is really important that your doctor checks the protein in your urine every year. When you have protein in your urine, it is a sign of kidney disease and kidney failure, and kidney disease is one of the most serious diabetes complications. If you have protein in your urine, there is evidence that if you cut back on the protein in your diet, then you may reduce your risk of developing kidney disease.

Many of the low-carbohydrate fad diets that keep you off carbohydrates and raise the amount of protein you eat cause me and anyone who cares about people with diabetes to be concerned. If you're eating so much protein, you may be increasing the risk of developing kidney disease. So, sure, you love burgers and steaks, but are they worth losing your kidneys and dying? Protecting your kidneys is important, and you will probably want to choose alternative protein foods, such as nuts and vegetables, to improve your dietary safety.

There is some thought in the diabetes community that protein intake makes the pancreas produce insulin in patients who have type 2 diabetes and are still producing insulin. If the body makes more insulin than it uses, the chance of insulin resistance is a real problem. Remember also that the more insulin you take, the harder it is to lose weight. So here's another reason to reduce your protein intake: if you make more insulin, you might become more insulin resistant, and then you may gain weight and/or your diabetes will get harder to manage.

For patients who experience overnight hypoglycemia, some care providers recommend eating a food higher in protein and fat before bed, which will slowly raise your blood sugar during the night to prevent nighttime low blood sugar episodes, and recommend long-acting food bars as your bedtime snack.

Fat

Well, fats are what get us in trouble. Foods that contain a lot of fat or are cooked in fat are the junk we crave. Here's a short list of some tasty fatty foods: ice cream, chocolate candy, cookies, pies, cakes, chips, fried chicken, French fries, and pizza. This list could go on and on and on. Did I list a lot of your favorite foods? I am sure I did. Let's just

Not only will you need to pay attention to how much fat and the kinds of fats that are in the foods you buy and prepare, but you'll also have to watch out for "added fats," which we add while cooking. Many of us add fat to foods in order to add more taste and flavor. I don't need to tell you what these added fats are because you're probably already very familiar with them, but here's a short list anyway: butter, oil, and lard. You should watch for these added fats like a hawk. Taking healthy foods and adding fat to them when cooking is a terrible way to manage your meal plan.

Here's an example. Let's say you're eating some healthy broccoli.

Here is the nutritional information for 3 1/2 ounces of broccoli:

Nutrition Facts

Amount Per Serving

Calories 22	Calories from Fat 5

Total Fat 0.5g

Saturated Fat 0.1g

Cholesterol 0mg

Sodium 33mg

Total Carbohydrate 2.8g

Dietary Fiber 2.7g

Sugars 0.3g

Protein 3.2g

Calories per gram:
Fat 9 • Carbohydrate 4 • Protein 4

admit it, fatty foods taste good, and they are often the comfort food we crave when we are tired, stressed, sad, or depressed. They often carried over from childhood, and these foods bring back memories of the easier, better times in your life, often before you were diagnosed with diabetes.

There are different kinds of fats, but whichever you choose to include in your meal, they need to be measured and counted. Fats should constitute the smallest portion of your meal plan because they pack in the most calories per gram of food. This, of course, can lead to weight gain, clogged arteries, and other conditions that may badly affect

And then, to top it all off, you cook it in what you think is just a tiny bit (one tablespoon) of butter or margarine. Take a look at the table below and add those details to the nutrient data above and look how you've changed just a small serving of broccoli.

Product (per 1 Tbsp)	Calories	Total fat (grams)	Saturated fat (grams)	Trans fat (grams)	Cholesterol (mg)
Butter	102	11	7	0.5	31
Margarine (stick)	80–100	9–11	1–2	1–3	0
Margarine (soft)	5–102	0–12	0–4	0–2.5	12

Do you see? Under the best circumstances, you've added at least five calories to the serving if you used the lightest, healthiest soft margarine on the market. But, if you instead went with the butter, your serving of broccoli packs a wallop: 124 calories, 11.5 grams of fat, 7.1 grams of saturated fat, 0.5 gram of trans fat, and 31 mg of cholesterol. The fats and cholesterol weren't even in the original food! So please, do yourself a favor and avoid adding fats to your meals.

your health. Now, let's break down the fats into their different types, so you know what you're actually reading about when you look at a food label.

Saturated Fats

The most common sources of saturated fats are foods from animals, whole-milk dairy products, lard, and oils, such as coconut and palm oils. Saturated fats raise your cholesterol levels, which is not healthy, and are found in all of those foods you love but shouldn't be eating, such as cheeseburgers, snack chips, crackers, cakes, and pastries. As you can probably tell, they make foods taste really good. So, like a lot of advice, it's easier to say it than to do it, but you're going to have to cut down on these foods and try to cut them out of your meal plan when possible. Whenever possible, try to substitute the saturated fats in your diet with foods that contain polyunsaturated or monounsaturated fats.

Trans Fats

Cities have started banning trans fats, so you've probably heard of them by now. But what are these mysterious new fats? Trans fats are produced when liquid oil is made into a solid fat. This process is called hydrogenation. Trans fats act like saturated fats and can raise your cholesterol level. Trans fats are now listed on food labels, making it easier to identify and avoid these foods. Keep in mind that if there is a 0.5 gram or less of trans fat in a food, the label can claim zero grams. If you want to avoid as much trans fat as possible, you must read the ingredient list on food labels. Look for words like hydrogenated oil or partially hydrogenated oil. Select foods that do not contain hydrogenated oil or in which liquid oil is listed first in the ingredient list. Here are some common sources of trans fat.

- Processed foods such as snacks (crackers and chips) and baked goods (muffins, cookies and cakes) that are made with hydrogenated oil or partially hydrogenated oil
- Stick margarines
- Shortening
- Some fast food items, such as French fries

Monounsaturated Fats

Monounsaturated fats are "healthy" fats. They can lower your "bad" (LDL, or low-density lipoprotein) cholesterol and are the fats I most recommend for a healthy diet. Not only are they good for you, but they also taste good! Sources of monounsaturated fat include:

- Avocado
- Canola oil
- Nuts, such as almonds, cashews, pecans, and peanuts
- Olive oil and olives
- Peanut butter and peanut oil
- Sesame seeds

To include more monounsaturated fats in your diet, try to substitute olive or canola oil instead of butter, margarine, or shortening when cooking. Sprinkling a few nuts or sesame seeds on a salad is an easy way to eat more monounsaturated fats. But be careful! Nuts and oils are high in calories, like all fats. If you are trying to lose or maintain your weight, you want to eat small portions of these foods. For example, 6 almonds or 4 pecan halves have the same number of calories as 1 teaspoon of oil or butter. Work with your dietitian to include healthy fats in your meal plan without increasing your total calories.

Polyunsaturated Fats

These fats are a "healthier" fat. Polyunsaturated fats have been shown to lower cholesterol levels, but may not be great for your healthy (HDL, or high-density lipoprotein) cholesterol levels. You may choose to include these in your diet as well as monounsaturated fats. You can find polyunsaturated fats in:

- Corn oil
- Cottonseed oil
- Safflower oil
- Soybean oil
- Sunflower oil
- Walnuts
- Pumpkin or sunflower seeds
- Soft tub margarine
- Mayonnaise
- Some salad dressings

Omega-3 Fatty Acids

Omega-3 fatty acids help prevent clogged arteries. Some types of fish are high in omega-3 fatty acids. You should eat non-fried fish two or three times a week. Not only will they not raise your "bad" cholesterol level, but they have been shown to reduce the risks of developing of coronary vascu-

Eat More Fish

I get teased all the time about how I gave up red meat and most foods with cholesterol, but I can't help it. Instead, I love sushi and eat lots of raw fish! It's easy for me because I live in the Florida Keys and I like to fish. But I'm sure I'm not the only one out there who enjoys eating fish, so here are some great recipes to get you started.

Baked Flounder au Gratin
Serves 4, Serving size: 3 oz

1 large flounder (about 2 lb)
Salt to taste (optional)
Juice of 1 lemon
¼ cup dried bread crumbs
¼ cup shredded, reduced-fat cheddar cheese
3 Tbsp reduced-fat margarine
½ cup minced onion

1. Have your fish dealer dress the fish for you, which means removing the scales, insides, head, and tail.
2. Heat the oven to 375°F. Sprinkle the fish with salt and lemon juice. Lay fish in shallow nonstick baking dish.
3. Cover with bread crumbs, cheese, small lumps of margarine, and onion. Bake for 35–45 minutes or until fish flakes easily when tested with a fork. Baste the fish from time to time with the pan juices.

Nutrition information: Calories 167, Calories from fat 55, Total fat 6 g, Saturated fat 1 g, Cholesterol 48 mg, Sodium 254 mg, Total carbohydrate 8 g, Dietary fiber 1 g, Sugars 2 g, Protein 19 g. Exchanges: 1/2 starch, 3 very lean meat, 1/2 fat.

From *The New Soul Food Cookbook for People with Diabetes, 2nd Edition,* by Fabiola Demps Gaines and Roniece Weaver.

Asian Tuna Steaks
Serves 6, Serving size: 3–4 oz

Marinade

¼ cup orange juice
  (fresh or frozen)
2 Tbsp sesame oil
2 tsp sesame seeds

3 Tbsp lite soy sauce
1 Tbsp fresh grated ginger
  (or 2 tsp ground ginger)
3 Tbsp chopped scallions

Tuna

1½ lb tuna steaks

1. In a stainless steel bowl or plastic zip-top bag, combine all marinade ingredients. Add the tuna and let it marinate for 20 minutes.
2. Broil or grill the tuna 6 inches from the heat source for 4–5 minutes per side. Cook until done as desired (some people prefer their tuna more rare than others do).

Nutrition information: Calories 184, Calories from fat 71, Total fat 8 g, Saturated fat 2 g, Cholesterol 42 mg, Sodium 194 mg, Total carbohydrate 1 g, Dietary fiber 0 g, Sugars 1 g, Protein 26 g. Exchanges: 3 lean meat.

From *Diabetic Meals in 30 Minutes—Or Less!, 2nd Edition,* by Robyn Webb.

Cajun Halibut
Serves 4,
Serving Size: 1 halibut steak

¼ tsp salt
1 tsp black pepper
¼ tsp ground red pepper

¼ tsp paprika
¼ tsp garlic powder
4 halibut steaks (4 ounces each)

1. In a small bowl, combine the salt, black and ground red peppers, paprika, and garlic powder; mix well. Rub evenly over both sides of the fish.
2. Preheat a large nonstick skillet over medium-high heat. When hot, remove from the heat and, away from the cooking surface, coat with nonstick cooking spray.
3. Return the skillet to the heat, add the fish, and cook for 3–4 minutes per side, or until the fish is cooked through and flakes easily with a fork. Serve immediately.

Nutrition information: Calories 126, Calories from fat 23, Total fat 3 g, Saturated fat 0 g, Cholesterol 37 mg, Sodium 208 mg, Total carbohydrate 0 g, Dietary fiber 0 g, Sugars 0 g, Protein 24 g. Exchanges: 4 very lean meat.

From *Mr. Food's Quick & Easy Diabetic Cooking,* by Art Ginsburg.

Often, fish gets a bad reputation for having too much cholesterol, so here is a list of common fish and their nutritional
values and cholesterol levels.

Fish	Serving size	Calories	Carbs (g)	Fat (g)	% Cal. from fat	Sat. fat (g)	Cholesterol (mg)	Sodium (mg)	Fiber (g)	Protein (g)
Cod	3 oz	89	0	1	10	0	47	66	0	19
Flounder/ Sole	3 oz	99	0	1	14	0	58	89	0	21
Haddock	3 oz	95	0	1	7	0	63	74	0	21
Halibut	3 oz	119	0	2	19	0	35	59	0	23
Mackerel, King	3 oz	114	0	2	18	0	58	173	0	22
Rainbow Trout	3 oz	144	0	6	38	2	58	36	0	21
Salmon, Atlantic/ Coho	3 oz	175	0	10	54	2	54	52	0	19
Sea Bass	3 oz	105	0	2	19	0	45	74	0	20
Tuna, Yellowfin	3 oz	118	0	1	8	0	49	40	0	25

From *The Diabetes Carbohydrate & Fat Gram Guide,* by Lea Ann Holzmeister.

lar disease, which is a kind of heart disease. You can find
omega-3 fatty acids in:

- Albacore tuna
- Herring
- Mackerel
- Rainbow trout
- Sardines
- Salmon

Some plant foods are also sources of omega-3 fatty
acids. These sources include:

- Tofu and other soybean products
- Walnuts
- Flaxseed and flaxseed oil
- Canola oil

Cholesterol

We know that people with diabetes have a higher risk of heart
disease than people without diabetes and that cholesterol levels are directly related to putting people at even higher risk of

Just so you don't forget, here's a list of fats that is broken down into what you should choose often and what you should try to reduce or avoid.

Choose often:	Choose occasionally or try to avoid:
▪ olive oil	
▪ canola oil	▪ butter
▪ peanut oil	▪ cream cheese
▪ avocados	▪ hydrogenated oil
▪ safflower oil	▪ trans fats
▪ nuts	▪ sour cream
▪ corn oil	▪ red meats
▪ soybean oil	▪ skin of poultry
▪ sesame oil	

developing heart disease. The American Heart Association and the American Diabetes Association have joined forces in a major campaign to encourage the American public to be aware of and reduce your intake of cholesterol.

GROCERY SHOPPING

Let's talk about grocery shopping. After all, you need to buy healthy foods to power a healthy meal plan. In all of my classes, I give my patients and colleagues a fun tip about shopping. When you go to a supermarket, shop around the walls of the store. What does that mean? Well, if you look at a store, the real foods that need refrigeration are around the walls, so they can plug in the refrigerators and keep the food cool. Foods that can spoil or rot are foods that have not been overly processed or loaded with additives, so in general, they will be healthier. The meats, vegetables, dairy, fish, fruits, and other great-tasting stuff are around the edges of your grocery store. Processed and canned package foods that will live for-

ever tend to be in the middle of the store, surrounded by
cleaning products, paper plates, and party goods.

This may be simplified, but it's a tip that works if you
use your knowledge when shopping. There are exceptions,
however; a can of sardines or salmon is healthier for you
than that ten-layer cake in the bakery. Whole-wheat pasta
is healthier than regular sour cream. Just remember, when
you shop the walls, go lean with the meats, choose nonfat
with the dairy, and avoid those pastries. You'll do fine if
you start with that little bit of knowledge. The best tip I can
give you is next: read your food labels.

Reading Food Labels

Label A

Nutrition Facts

Serving Size 1 cup (228g)
Servings Per Container 2

Amount Per Serving

Calories 260   Calories from Fat 120

	% Daily Value*
Total Fat 13g	20%
Saturated Fat 5g	25%
Trans Fat 2g	
Cholesterol 30mg	10%
Sodium 660mg	28%
Total Carbohydrate 31g	10%
Dietary Fiber 0g	0%
Sugars 5g	
Protein 5g	

Vitamin A 4%	•	Vitamin C 2%
Calcium 15%	•	Iron 4%

*Percent Daily Values are based on a 2,000
calorie diet. Your Daily Values may be higher or
lower depending on your calorie needs.

	Calories:	2,000	2,500
Total Fat	Less than	65g	80g
Sat Fat	Less than	20g	25g
Cholesterol	Less than	300mg	300mg
Sodium	Less than	2,400mg	2,400mg
Total Carbohydrate		300g	375g
Dietary Fiber		25g	30g

Calories per gram:
Fat 9 • Carbohydrate 4 • Protein 4

One of the most important skills you can learn when shopping for food (or eating out) is how to read a food label. All foods sold in the U.S. must be labeled and follow the guidelines of the U.S. Food and Drug Administration. Food labels explain everything you need to know, so you can decide whether you should eat that food. It makes a lot of sense to eat a snack that has less than 7 grams of fat instead of potato chips that have 11 grams of fat, but there's more to reading food labels than just looking at the fat grams. Let me show you what is on a label and what you should be looking at.

Let's look at this label (Label A). When looking at a food label, you should always ask yourself, "Is this food worth it?"

1. Look at the serving size and number of servings on Label A. Notice that the package contains two servings. So, this pretty small package contains two cups in it, and you should only eat half of it per serving. If you eat the entire package, you need to double all of the nutrition information.

2. Look at the amount of total calories in Label A. It says it contains 260 calories. But if you eat the entire package, then you've just eaten 520 calories. Wow! That's about one-third of what a person should usually eat in a day.

3. Look at the fat content in Label A. It has 13 grams of total fat. Five grams of that comes from saturated fat and 2 grams from trans fat. We want to avoid this much fat and these specific kinds of fats.

4. There are 31 grams of carbohydrate and no dietary fiber to slow that absorption down. That's a lot of carbohydrate for a snack.

5. If you're watching your blood pressure, like I do, then you'll also need to take into account the food's sodium content. A dietitian will be able to help you here if that's your case.

6. Label A is for a cereal. You might want to make another choice. Look at Label B and compare.

Label B

Nutrition Facts

Serving Size 30g

Amount Per Serving

Calories 78   Calories from Fat 13

	% Daily Value*
Total Fat 1g	**2%**
Saturated Fat 0g	**1%**
Trans Fat 0g	
Cholesterol 0mg	**0%**
Sodium 73mg	**3%**
Total Carbohydrate 22g	**7%**
Dietary Fiber 9g	**35%**
Sugars 5g	
Protein 4g	

Vitamin A 10%	•	Vitamin C 10%
Calcium 12%	•	Iron 29%

*Percent Daily Values are based on a 2,000 calorie diet. Your Daily Values may be higher or lower depending on your calorie needs.

	Calories:	2,000	2,500
Total Fat	Less than	65g	80g
Sat Fat	Less than	20g	25g
Cholesterol	Less than	300mg	300mg
Sodium	Less than	2,400mg	2,400mg
Total Carbohydrate		300g	375g
Dietary Fiber		25g	30g

Calories per gram:

Fat 9 • Carbohydrate 4 • Protein 4

MAKING SMART CHOICES IN RESTAURANTS

Eating out is an important and fun part of our lives and should not be excluded from your life simply because you have diabetes. All it will take is some planning and careful reading of menus. You'll need to consult with your health care providers to learn how you should plan and adjust your medications before you eat out. Also, you may need to adjust your daily meals around your plans for eating out. A lot of this requires that you speak directly with your dietitian and doctors, so I can't help you there. But I can teach you to read menus with a health-conscious eye.

Reading menus can be an exciting and fun experience and not just because of all of the foods that you want to eat. When you first start looking at menus with a health-conscious eye, you might be surprised by your new outlook on food selection. Menus are so difficult when you're looking for those healthy, wholesome choices, especially when the menu is huge. Sometimes I can barely lift the menu at some restaurants because there are so many choices.

Here are four excellent tips for tackling menus and eating out. They should help you deal with the cultural idea that we need to finish everything on our plates. This gets us into so much trouble. Did your mother tell you that? I remember my mother telling me that kids in Europe were starving and I was wasting food, even though she never sent my leftovers anywhere. The other thing we do is pick at the food on our plates after we are satisfied and full. If there is food on the plate after we're done eating, the temptation to eat a little more is always there. If the food is out of sight, then it is out of mind and you won't eat it. Following these tips will cut down on the amount of food you will actually eat.

Remember, meals don't have to be a burden or a problem. They should be a normal part of your life.

#1: You Don't Need to Clean Your Plate

Remember, it is acceptable to order a food and only eat half of it. You can take home the leftovers. Even more, you can just leave it behind to be cleared away. Get the old idea that you can't waste food out of your head. It drives me crazy! It doesn't make sense, because if you do keep eating whatever you want, your diabetes will become more difficult to manage and you'll eventually end up shortening your life.

Keep this in mind: it is always acceptable to share a main course. Restaurants have made a killing by giving us more food than any one person should ever eat in a single meal, and it keeps us coming back for more. Don't fall into their trap, and follow my advice: split that entrée with a buddy. Order an extra salad or soup and share the main dish with your eating partner. Doing this will not only save you calories or carbohydrates, but it will also save you money.

#2: Appetizers Can Be Your Friend

Think about just ordering two appetizers for you and your eating partner. Usually, one appetizer is enough for one person. The appetizers in some restaurants are a full portion, and try to stay away from those sampler-sized appetizers that give you a little bit of everything. Those really are big enough for two people! If you share an appetizer or two with your meal companion, you can each order a side salad. Surprise! You now have a great and relatively healthy meal. I actually prefer to eat these appetizer meals because I get to taste different things, which is always fun.

#3: Order a To-Go Box with Your Meal

Here's a great one for those times when no one wants to share with you or when you're eating by yourself. When

you get your main course, ask for a take-out box immediately. Put half of the meal in the box, put it out of sight,
and enjoy the rest. Enjoy the leftovers as another meal.

#4: Get Help from a Dietitian

The most important tip I can give you is to make an
appointment with a dietitian. They are wonderful people
and should be a major part of your support team. I'm not
going to stop telling you to see one, so you might as well
make that appointment right now.

A Fun Exercise

In the next series of pages, you will see five menus from
restaurants from different cultures and with different types
of food. For each menu, select everything you would choose
to eat for one meal: breakfast, lunch, or dinner. At the end
of this chapter will be the same menu, but I will have
selected certain healthy items to order. These may be items
you did not choose or think of as a healthy alternative.

As a demonstration, I'll go through the first one with
you. This is a very simple menu from a Greek restaurant
that would be found in most cities and towns around the
country. Because eating in a restaurant is a treat, you probably don't want to choose something that you can cook at
home. So let's start with the appetizers.

Appetizers

There are seven items to choose from. First, eliminate the
things you don't like at all and it will cut down the choices.
So, if you hate clams, then you're already down to five
items to choose from.

If you do not know what is in a menu item, ask your server. He or she will tell you what it is and how it is made.

If you are keeping an eye on your cholesterol as well as the fat calories in meals you should also avoid the fried appetizers, such as calamari or fried mozzarella sticks. Did you know that most calamari dishes are fried? If you didn't, then you should ask your server.

Now you can choose from the shrimp, stuffed artichoke hearts, and stuffed mushroom caps. Stuffing often means bread, so ask if the stuffing is mostly seafood or mostly bread.

This sounds like a lot of work, doesn't it? Don't worry. Once you get used to it and do this a few times, it'll become second nature.

Soups and Salads

Let's look at the soups and salads. Salads are always wonderful but not when they come loaded with cheeses or heavy dressings. So find out what is in the salad by reading the menu carefully or asking your server. Try adding some fruit to it instead of hard-boiled eggs or lots of cheese. Ask what light dressings are available or try a little olive oil and vinegar instead. Many people use lemon juice as a dressing, and this is a great, healthy option. You should always ask for the dressing on the side, too. That way, you get to decide how much dressing goes on and not the chef.

Soups are wonderful, especially on cold days, but you need to think healthy when you choose soup. You don't really want thick, creamy soups because they have too much fat, calories, cholesterol, and so forth. It is usually better to choose a vegetable-based soup or a broth-based soup with vegetables. For example, try choosing Manhattan clam chowder over New England clam chowder. Manhattan clam chowder has a tomato and vegetable stock, whereas the New England version has a cream base.

Main Courses
Now you're at the entrées or main courses. If you don't recognize the Greek food, find out which items are broiled or baked and which are fried. Which one contains sausage? Which one has plain beef or chicken? Cooking methods count, so be sure you find out about these things.

At this restaurant, you will also be offered side dishes. Two vegetables are always a great choice for side dishes. Try that instead of one vegetable and another side with rice or spaghetti. I'm going to have to burst some bubbles here, but potatoes are not considered vegetables. When healthy eating is concerned, you need to get your potatoes baked instead of fried, and if you do go for a baked potato, you're going to have to skip the sour cream, cheese, and butter. Even better, you might ask if you can only have one side. Portion sizes in restaurants are often too big.

The tip we used for salad dressing works well for gravies also. Ask for your gravy on the side. You might also try au jus gravy instead; it is a thin natural juice instead of heavy, thickened gravy. Salsa can perk up a meal and is low in calories and cholesterol, too.

Desserts
Desserts are not on this part of the menu, but we know that it's always a challenge skipping dessert or even choosing a healthy one. However, you can have dessert if you choose foods that are lower in calories and are still flavorful. Fresh fruit is always a great choice, and angel food cake is a lot better for you than a banana cream pie. A little ice cream is fine sometimes, but the whole bowl is often not an option because it can have as many calories as your entire meal. When I dine with friends, we order one dessert and everyone gets a fork to share it. We love doing this and get to leave the guilt at home because it was good and good for us.

Now, Try It Yourself!

I hope that this exercise will give you a jumpstart on making healthy choices at a restaurant. You can always get more help from your dietitian or diabetes educator. Look through the other menus and try to make healthy choices, and then turn to the menus that I have marked up, showing healthy selections. Are you surprised by some of my choices? If you are, then bring these to your health care team and maybe they can give you some more tips. You might want to copy these menus and ask your family and friends to think about what they would choose. Make this a fun game. As I said, this is just a starting point, but you're going to have to do this on your own in the future, so getting started now will put you in a great place for moving forward in the future.

Don't lose hope! More and more restaurants are doing you a favor by noting healthy choices on their menus. They often call them "healthy choices" and that can be very helpful when you are making decisions. When you're lucky enough to have a menu like this, just pretend that the other items without this notation don't exist. You've already cut out more than half of the menu!

Food should not be a burden. It is a part of life, and I hope the knowledge you now have will make you feel more comfortable and less overwhelmed. There are lots of people out there to help you and wonderful books and references.

EL GRECO CAFE

APPETIZERS

Clams Casino	7.95
Shrimp Cocktail	7.95
Fried Mozzarella Sticks (homemade)	5.50
Steamed Clams (one dozen w/ drawn butter)	8.95
Stuffed Artichoke Hearts with Seafood	5.95
Stuffed Mushroom Caps with Seafood	5.50
Fried Calamari (with marinara sauce for dipping)	6.50

SOUPS AND SALADS

Crock of French Onion Soup			3.50
Soup Du Jour	Cup......2.50	Bowl 3.25	
Fresh Garden Salad			5.95
Greek Salad			8.95
Antipasto Salad			8.95
Caesar Salad			8.95
With Grilled Chicken		add	4.00

GREEK SPECIALTIES

Spanakopita with Greek Salad	10.95
Moussaka with Greek Salad	10.95
Gyro Platter with Greek Salad	10.95
Grilled Chicken or Pork Shish ke bab	13.95
With Tomatoes, Onion & Peppers over Rice	

ENTREES

Includes a cup of soup or salad (house, Greek or antipasto), rice and vegetable or pasta

Veal Alla Athens	15.95
Veal and Eggplant Parmigiana with Linguini	
Veal-Marsala, Francaise or Piccata	13.95
Veal Parmigiana with Linguini	13.95

PASTA

Includes cup of soup or salad (house, Greek or antipasto)

Penne AlaVodka	11.95
Prosciutto and Peas in a Vodka Pink Sauce	
Penne Siciliano	11.95
Plum Tomato Sauce with Eggplant, Onions, Garlic and Basil	
Linguini with Red or White Clam Sauce	10.95
Linguini with Marinara Sauce	9.95
Linguini with Olive Oil and Garlic	10.95
Fettucini Alfredo	9.95

EL GRECO CAFE

APPETIZERS

Clams Casino	7.95
Shrimp Cocktail	7.95
Fried Mozzarella Sticks (homemade)	5.50
Steamed Clams (one dozen w/ drawn butter)	8.95
Stuffed Artichoke Hearts with Seafood	5.95
Stuffed Mushroom Caps with Seafood	5.50
Fried Calamari (with marinara sauce for dipping)	6.50

SOUPS AND SALADS

Crock of French Onion Soup			3.50
Soup Du Jour	Cup......2.50	Bowl.....3.25	
Fresh Garden Salad			5.95
Greek Salad			8.95
Antipasto Salad			8.95
Caesar Salad			8.95
With Grilled Chicken		add	4.00

GREEK SPECIALTIES

Spanakopita with Greek Salad	10.95
Moussaka with Greek Salad	10.95
Gyro Platter with Greek Salad	10.95
Grilled Chicken or Pork Shish ke bab	13.95
With Tomatoes, Onion & Peppers over Rice	

ENTREES

Includes a cup of soup or salad (house, Greek or antipasto), rice and vegetable or pasta

Veal Alla Athens	15.95
Veal and Eggplant Parmigiana with Linguini	
Veal-Marsala, Francaise or Piccata	13.95
Veal Parmigiana with Linguini	13.95

PASTA

Includes cup of soup or salad (house, Greek or antipasto)

Penne Ala Vodka	11.95
Prosciutto and Peas in a Vodka Pink Sauce	
Penne Siciliano	11.95
Plum Tomato Sauce with Eggplant, Onions, Garlic and Basil	
Linguini with Red or White Clam Sauce	10.95
Linguini with Marinara Sauce	9.95
Linguini with Olive Oil and Garlic	10.95
Fettucini Alfredo	9.95

HUNAN DYNASTY

PORK

M23.	Moo Shu Pork *(Served w. 4 Pancakes)*	8.25
M24.	Hunan Pork	8.25
M25.	Roast Pork w. Chinese Vegetable	8.25
M26.	Twice Cooked Pork	8.25
M27.	Pork w. Garlic Sauce	8.25
M28.	Spareribs w. Black Bean Sauce	8.95

NOODLE

M29.	Vegetable, Roast Pork or Chicken Chow Fun	6.95
M30.	Vegetable, Roast Pork or Chicken Rice Noodle	6.95
M31.	Beef or Shrimp Chow Fun	7.50
M32.	Beef or Shrimp Rice Noodle	7.50
M33.	Singapore Rice Noodle	8.50
M34.	Vegetable, Chicken or Roast Pork Lo Mein or Chow Mein	6.95
M35.	Beef or Shrimp Lo Mein or Chow Mein	7.50
M36.	House Special Lo Mein or Chow Mein	8.50

FRIED RICE

M37.	Vegetable, Chicken or Roast Pork Fried Rice	6.45
M38.	Beef or Shrimp Fried Rice	7.50
M39.	Hunan Dynasty's Fried Rice	8.50

SEAFOOD

F 1.	Shrimp w. Broccoli	10.45
F 2.	Shrimp w. Cashew Nuts	10.45
F 3.	Kung Pao Shrimp w. Peanut	10.45
F 4.	Moo Shu Shrimp *(Served w. 4 Pancakes)*	10.45
F 5.	Shrimp Szechuan Style	10.45
F 6.	Sweet & Sour Shrimp	10.45
F 7.	Shrimp w. Garlic Sauce	10.45
F 8.	Shrimp w. Lobster Sauce	10.45
F 9.	Shrimp w. Snow Peas	11.45
F10.	Sizzling Seafood	13.95
F11.	Lobster Any Style	Seasonal
	Ginger & scallops, black bean sauce, garlic sauce, Szechuan & Cantonese.	
F12.	Peppery Calamari	9.95
F13.	Clams w. Black Bean Sauce	10.45
F14.	Stir-Fried Jumbo Shrimp	13.95

LIGHT & HEALTHY

Stir-Fried w. Light Sauce, No Corn Starch, Less Oil, Low in Salt & Sugar.

D 1.	Mixed Vegetables in Spicy Basil Seasoning	8.45
D 2.	Chicken & Vegetable in Spicy Orange Sauce	9.45
D 3.	Lemon Flavored Chicken & Vegetable	9.45
D 4.	Shrimp & Vegetable in Szechuan Sauce	10.95
D 5.	Scallop & Vegetable in Spicy Garlic Sauce	11.45

DIET SPECIALTIES

Steamed w. Light Brown Sauce or Ginger & Scallion Sauce on the Side. Served w. Brown Rice

D 6.	Chicken w. Mixed Vegetables	8.95
D 7.	Seafood Delight	13.95
D 8.	Chicken w. Broccoli	8.25
D 9.	Shrimp w. Mixed Vegetables	10.95
D10.	Buddhist Delight	8.25

VEGETABLE

V 1.	Moo Shu Vegetable *(Served w. 4 Pancakes)*	6.95
V 2.	Mixed Vegetable Delight	6.95
V 3.	Sauteed String Beans	6.95
V 4.	Eggplant w. Garlic Sauce	6.95
V 5.	Bean Curd Family Style	6.95
V 6.	Broccoli w. Garlic Sauce	6.95
V 7.	Spinach w. Fresh Garlic	7.95
V 8.	Peppery Crispy Bean Curd	7.95
V 9.	Buddhist Rolls Platter	9.95
V10.	Vegetarian Fried Brown Rice	9.95

VEGETARIAN CUISINE

All Dishes Made From Vegetable & Soy Bean Portion

V 1.	Vegetable Chicken w. Eggplant & Tofu	8.95
V 2.	Walnut Vegetable Chicken & String Bean	9.95
V 3.	Golden Sesame Bean Curd	8.95
V 4.	Tofu Delight w. Black Bean Sauce	8.95
V 5.	Vegetable Chicken w. Broccoli	8.95
V 6.	Curry Vegetable Chicken	8.95
V 7.	Golden Crispy Orange Vegetable Beef	10.95
V 8.	General Tso's Vegetable Chicken	10.95

HUNAN DYNASTY

PORK

M23.	Moo Shu Pork *(Served w. 4 Pancakes)*	8.25
M24.	Hunan Pork	8.25
M25.	Roast Pork w. Chinese Vegetable	8.25
M26.	Twice Cooked Pork	8.25
M27.	Pork w. Garlic Sauce	8.25
M28.	Spareribs w. Black Bean Sauce	8.95

NOODLE

M29.	Vegetable, Roast Pork or Chicken Chow Fun	6.95
M30.	Vegetable, Roast Pork or Chicken Rice Noodle	6.95
M31.	Beef or Shrimp Chow Fun	7.50
M32.	Beef or Shrimp Rice Noodle	7.50
M33.	Singapore Rice Noodle	8.50
M34.	Vegetable, Chicken or Roast Pork Lo Mein or Chow Mein	6.95
M35.	Beef or Shrimp Lo Mein or Chow Mein	7.50
M36.	House Special Lo Mein or Chow Mein	8.50

FRIED RICE

M37.	Vegetable, Chicken or Roast Pork Fried Rice	6.45
M38.	Beef or Shrimp Fried Rice	7.50
M39.	Hunan Dynasty's Fried Rice	8.50

SEAFOOD

F 1.	Shrimp w. Broccoli	10.45
F 2.	Shrimp w. Cashew Nuts	10.45
F 3.	Kung Pao Shrimp w. Peanut	10.45
F 4.	Moo Shu Shrimp *(Served w. 4 Pancakes)*	10.45
F 5.	Shrimp Szechuan Style	10.45
F 6.	Sweet & Sour Shrimp	10.45
F 7.	Shrimp w. Garlic Sauce	10.45
F 8.	Shrimp w. Lobster Sauce	10.45
F 9.	Shrimp w. Snow Peas	11.45
F10.	Sizzling Seafood	13.95
F11.	Lobster Any Style	Seasonal
	Ginger & scallops, black bean sauce,	
	garlic sauce, Szechuan & Cantonese.	
F12.	Peppery Calamari	9.95
F13.	Clams w. Black Bean Sauce	10.45
F14.	Stir-Fried Jumbo Shrimp	13.95

LIGHT & HEALTHY

Stir-Fried w. Light Sauce, No Corn Starch, Less Oil, Low in Salt & Sugar.

D 1.	Mixed Vegetables in Spicy Basil Seasoning	8.45
D 2.	Chicken & Vegetable in Spicy Orange Sauce	9.45
D 3.	Lemon Flavored Chicken & Vegetable	9.45
D 4.	Shrimp & Vegetable in Szechuan Sauce	10.95
D 5.	Scallop & Vegetable in Spicy Garlic Sauce	11.45

DIET SPECIALTIES

Steamed w. Light Brown Sauce or Ginger & Scallion Sauce on the Side. Served w. Brown Rice

D 6.	Chicken w. Mixed Vegetables	8.95
D 7.	Seafood Delight	13.95
D 8.	Chicken w. Broccoli	8.25
D 9.	Shrimp w. Mixed Vegetables	10.95
D10.	Buddhist Delight	8.25

VEGETABLE GREAT

V 1.	Moo Shu Vegetable *(Served w. 4 Pancakes)*	6.95
V 2.	Mixed Vegetable Delight	6.95
V 3.	Sauteed String Beans	6.95
V 4.	Eggplant w. Garlic Sauce	6.95
V 5.	Bean Curd Family Style	6.95
V 6.	Broccoli w. Garlic Sauce	6.95
V 7.	Spinach w. Fresh Garlic	7.95
V 8.	Peppery Crispy Bean Curd	7.95
V 9.	Buddhist Rolls Platter	9.95
V10.	Vegetarian Fried Brown Rice	9.95

VEGETARIAN CUISINE

All Dishes Made From Vegetable & Soy Bean Portion

V 1.	Vegetable Chicken w. Eggplant & Tofu	8.95
V 2.	Walnut Vegetable Chicken & String Bean	9.95
V 3.	Golden Sesame Bean Curd	8.95
V 4.	Tofu Delight w. Black Bean Sauce	8.95
V 5.	Vegetable Chicken w. Broccoli	8.95
V 6.	Curry Vegetable Chicken	8.95
V 7.	Golden Crispy Orange Vegetable Beef	10.95
V 8.	General Tso's Vegetable Chicken	10.95

AKIRA
Japanese Restaurant

Appetizers

1. **Ika sansai** $4.95
   Smoked squid mixed vegetable
2. **Tako su** $5.95
   Octopus & cucumber with light vinegar sauce
3. **Nigiri sushi** $5.95
   Tuna, salmon, white fish, yellow fish - 1 pc each
4. **Sashimi** $5.95
   Tuna, salmon, white fish - 2 pcs each
5. **Sunomono** $6.95
   Octopus, surf clam, shrimp, crab stick, cucumber
6. **Oshinko** $3.45
   Assorted pickled radish & vegetables
7. **Beef negimaki 6 pcs** $4.95
8. **Beef & crab maki 6 pcs** $4.95
9. **Shrimp vegetable shumai** $3.95
   Japanese shrimp 6 pcs & vegetable dumpling 6 pcs
10. **Gyoza** $3.95
    Shrimp or vegetable fried dumpling 6 pcs
11. **Shrimp tempura 2 pcs** $3.95
12. **Vegetable tempura** $3.95
    Assorted 4 pcs
13. **Edamame** $2.95
    Steamed soybean
14. **Fried tofu** $3.45
    Korean style fried soft tofu with special sauce with
    scallion and katsuo bushi sprinkled on top
15. **Ohitashi** $3.95
    Steamed spinach

Dinner specials

Hot entree
Choice white rice or brown rice

Gobdol bibimbob $12.95
Choice: beef / assorted seafood korean style dish served
on top of a big bowl of steamed rice in a hot stone pot
with korean chili paste and miso soup (korean style
bbqed beef or assorted seafood, spinach, squash,
soybean sprout, carrot, shitake mushroom, sauteed
chinese radish, egg custard)

Soondooboo $9.95
Choice: beef / seafood / vegetable / kimchi / combo
Korean style soft tofu broth served with steamed rice
(flavor: mild / hot & spicy)

Teriyaki dinner $12.95
Chicken

Teriyaki dinner $14.95
Salmon

Teriyaki dinner $16.95
Shrimp / beef / beef negi / seafood / eel broccoli,
potato, carrot & cabbage served with steamed rice,
miso soup, salad

Shrimp tempura dinner $15.95
Shrimp tempura 6 pcs, steamed rice, miso soup, salad

Vegetable tempura dinner $12.95
Assorted vegetable tempura 8 pcs, steamed rice,
miso soup, salad

Tempura combo dinner $16.95
Shrimp tempura 4 pcs, vegetable tempura 8 pcs,
rice, miso soup, salad

1. **Zap chaz** $13.95
   Sweet potato noodle with assorted vegetables choice of
   beef, shrimp
2. **Shrimp tempura udon with tuna roll** $13.95
   Japanese white flour noodle bowl served with tuna roll
   6 pcs (shrimp tempura 2 pcs, fried tofu, fish cake,
   assorted vegetables)
3. **Veggie tempura udon with cucumber roll**
   $11.95
   Japanese white flour noodle bowl served with cucumber
   roll 6 pcs (vegetable tempura 3 pcs, fried tofu, assorted
   vegetables)
4. **Yaki udon** $9.95
   Fen fly noodle with mixed chicken and vegetable
5. **Ten don** $15.95
   Assorted tempura on top of steamed rice
6. **Tekka don** $15.95
   Tuna sashimi on top of sushi rice
7. **Kiji don** $15.95
   Chicken teriyaki on top of steamed rice
8. **Unagi don** $15.95
   Broiled fresh water eel on top of steamed rice
9. **Whedupbob** $15.95
   Korean style sashimi dish, served on top of steamed rice
   with (tuna, salmon, white fish, lettuce, cucumber, apple,
   radish, pepper, seaweed powder, sesame seed, masago,
   sesame oil, spicy korean sauce), miso soup

Party platters

Roll platter (10 rolls) $39.95
California roll 2, boston roll 1, eel roll 1, yellowtail
roll 1, salmon skin roll 1, spicy tuna roll 1, tuna roll 1,
salmon roll 1, cucumber roll 1

Sushi & roll platter $79.95
(24 pcs of sushi & 10 rolls)
24 pieces of sushi (tuna, yellowtail, eel, salmon, shrimp,
white fish, squid, octopus, surf clam, tuna, flying fish
roe, salmon roe)
california roll 2, boston roll 1, eel roll 1, yellowtail
roll 1, salmon skin roll 1, spicy tuna roll 1, tuna roll 1,
salmon roll 1, cucumber roll 1

Sushi & sashimi platter $99.95
(24 pcs of sushi & 32 pcs of sashimi)
24 pieces of sushi (tuna, yellowtail, eel, salmon, shrimp,
white fish, squid, octopus, surf clam, tuna, flying fish
roe, salmon roe)
32 pieces of sashimi (chef's choice)

We practice HACCP (hazard analysis & critical control
point) from raw material purchase to fine food preparation,
which is recommended and regulated by Food and Drug
Administration

We make brown rice sushi & roll

AKIRA
Japanese Restaurant

Appetizers

1. Ika sansai	$4.95
Smoked squid mixed vegetable	
2. Tako su	$5.95
Octopus & cucumber with light vinegar sauce	
3. Nigiri sushi	$5.95
Tuna, salmon, white fish, yellow fish - 1 pc each	
4. Sashimi	$5.95
Tuna, salmon, white fish - 2 pcs each	
5. Sunomono	$6.95
Octopus, surf clam, shrimp, crab stick, cucumber	
6. Oshinko	$3.45
Assorted pickled radish & vegetables	
7. Beef negimaki 6 pcs	$4.95
8. Beef & crab maki 6 pcs	$4.95
9. Shrimp vegetable shumai	$3.95
Japanese shrimp 6 pcs & vegetable dumpling 6 pcs	
10. Gyoza	$3.95
Shrimp or vegetable fried dumpling 6 pcs	
11. Shrimp tempura 2 pcs	$3.95
12. Vegetable tempura	$3.95
Assorted 4 pcs	
13. Edamame	$2.95
Steamed soybean	
14. Fried tofu	$3.45
Korean style fried soft tofu with special sauce with scallion and katsuo bushi sprinkled on top	
15. Ohitashi	$3.95
Steamed spinach	

Dinner specials

Hot entree
Choice white rice or brown rice

Gobdol bibimbob	$12.95

Choice: beef / assorted seafood korean style dish served on top of a big bowl of steamed rice in a hot stone pot with korean chili paste and miso soup (korean style bbqed beef or assorted seafood, spinach, squash, soybean sprout, carrot, shitake mushroom, sauteed chinese radish, egg custard)

Soondooboo	$9.95

Choice: beef / seafood / vegetable / kimchi / combo Korean style soft tofu broth served with steamed rice (flavor: mild / hot & spicy)

Teriyaki dinner	$12.95
Chicken	
Teriyaki dinner	$14.95
Salmon	
Teriyaki dinner	$16.95

Shrimp / beef / beef negi / seafood / eel broccoli, potato, carrot & cabbage served with steamed rice, miso soup, salad

Shrimp tempura dinner	$15.95
Shrimp tempura 6 pcs, steamed rice, miso soup, salad	
Vegetable tempura dinner	$12.95
Assorted vegetable tempura 8 pcs, steamed rice, miso soup, salad	
Tempura combo dinner	$16.95
Shrimp tempura 4 pcs, vegetable tempura 8 pcs, rice, miso soup, salad	

1. Zap chaz	$13.95
Sweet potato noodle with assorted vegetables choice of beef, shrimp	
2. Shrimp tempura udon with tuna roll	$13.95
Japanese white flour noodle bowl served with tuna roll 6 pcs (shrimp tempura 2 pcs, fried tofu, fish cake, assorted vegetables)	
3. Veggie tempura udon with cucumber roll	$11.95
Japanese white flour noodle bowl served with cucumber roll 6 pcs (vegetable tempura 3 pcs, fried tofu, assorted vegetables)	
4. Yaki udon	$9.95
Fen fly noodle with mixed chicken and vegetable	
5. Ten don	$15.95
Assorted tempura on top of steamed rice	
6. Tekka don	$15.95
Tuna sashimi on top of sushi rice	
7. Kiji don	$15.95
Chicken teriyaki on top of steamed rice	
8. Unagi don	$15.95
Broiled fresh water eel on top of steamed rice	
9. Whedupbob	$15.95
Korean style sashimi dish, served on top of steamed rice with (tuna, salmon, white fish, lettuce, cucumber, apple, radish, pepper, seaweed powder, sesame seed, masago, sesame oil, spicy korean sauce), miso soup	

Party platters

Roll platter (10 rolls)	$39.95

California roll 2, boston roll 1, eel roll 1, yellowtail roll 1, salmon skin roll 1, spicy tuna roll 1, tuna roll 1, salmon roll 1, cucumber roll 1

Sushi & roll platter	$79.95

(24 pcs of sushi & 10 rolls)
24 pieces of sushi (tuna, yellowtail, eel, salmon, shrimp, white fish, squid, octopus, surf clam, tuna, flying fish roe, salmon roe)
california roll 2, boston roll 1, eel roll 1, yellowtail roll 1, salmon skin roll 1, spicy tuna roll 1, tuna roll 1, salmon roll 1, cucumber roll 1

Sushi & sashimi platter	$99.95

(24 pcs of sushi & 32 pcs of sashimi)
24 pieces of sushi (tuna, yellowtail, eel, salmon, shrimp, white fish, squid, octopus, surf clam, tuna, flying fish roe, salmon roe)
32 pieces of sashimi (chef's choice)

We practice HACCP (hazard analysis & critical control point) from raw material purchase to fine food preparation, which is recommended and regulated by Food and Drug Administration

We make brown rice sushi & roll

La Bonita Grill

BURRITO BAR MENU $5.89
Create Yourself!

Burrito Muy Grande! It's Big!
Giant flour tortilla, cilantro lime or brown rice, choice of vegetarian black bean or pinto, choice of meat, choice of salsa, cheese or sour cream.

Burrito Fajita
Like the burrito but with freshly grilled peppers and onions instead of beans.

Naked Burrito
Burrito or fajita in a bowl, no tortilla. We add romaine lettuce, no rice.

WITH

Chicken	Pork	Ground Beef	Steak	Vegetarian
Hormone free skinless chicken breast, marinated over night, and chargrilled to perfection.	Shredded pork, seasoned and marinated then braised for hours.	Lean ground beef, seasoned with our spices and gently cooked to perfection.	Lean, marinated overnight and chargrilled.	Includes fresh-made guacamole & vegetarian beans, grilled peppers and onions.

Enchiladas
Two corn tortillas, chicken, steak, pork or cheese, topped with enchilada sauce and served with rice and beans.
Chicken, steak or pork $6.89   **Cheese** $6.59

Quesadilla
Melted jack cheese in a grilled flour tortilla with guacamole, sour cream & fresh pico de gallo on the side $4.89
Chicken, steak or pork quesadilla   add $1.89   **Vegetarian style**   add $1.29

SALAD

Bonita Tostada $5.45	Bonita Ensalada $6.89	Nachos $5.39
Romaine in a large crisp tortilla shell, topped with black beans, tomato, cheese, guacamole, sour cream & homemade vinaigrette dressing. **With chicken, steak or pork add $1.85**	Marinated, chargrilled chicken tossed with crisp romaine lettuce, crispy tortilla strips, pico de gallo, olive oil vinaigrette dressing, tossed to order and topped with shaved cheese	Tortilla chips covered with melted jack and cheddar cheese, black beans, sour cream, guacamole and fresh pico de gallo **Try it with chicken, pork or steak add $1.19**

TACOS

Warm flour tortillas, stuffed with jack cheese, diced tomatoes and lettuce.

Taco Meal
Any 3 of our tacos. Chicken, steak or pork.
Served with a side of guacamole $5.89

Individual Taco
Charbroiled Steak	$2.65
Marinated Chicken	$2.65
Braised Pork	$2.65
Ground Beef	$2.65
Vegetarian	$2.50
(black beans, peppers & onions)

SIDE ORDERS

Chips		$1.89
Guacamole	**Small**	$1.89
Guacamole 8 oz side w/chips		$4.29
Fresh salsa made fresh daily 8 oz		$1.89
Rice or Beans (pinto or black)		$1.89
Sour Cream		$0.50

FAJITAS

Platter of charbroiled chicken, steak or pork grilled peppers, onions, rice, beans, sour cream and guacamole.
Corn or flour tortillas $7.95

La Bonita Grill

BURRITO BAR MENU $5.89
Create Yourself!

Burrito Muy Grande! It's Big!
Giant flour tortilla, cilantro lime or brown rice, choice of vegetarian black bean or pinto, choice of meat, choice of salsa, cheese or sour cream.

Burrito Fajita
Like the burrito but with freshly grilled peppers and onions instead of beans.

Naked Burrito
Burrito or fajita in a bowl, no tortilla. We add romaine lettuce, no rice.

WITH

Chicken	**Pork**	**Ground Beef**	**Steak**	**Vegetarian**
Hormone free skinless chicken breast, marinated over night, and chargrilled to perfection.	Shredded pork, seasoned and marinated then braised for hours.	Lean ground beef, seasoned with our spices and gently cooked to perfection.	Lean, marinated overnight and chargrilled.	Includes fresh-made guacamole & vegetarian beans, grilled peppers and onions.

Enchiladas
Two corn tortillas, chicken, steak, pork or cheese, topped with enchilada sauce and served with rice and beans.
Chicken, steak or pork $6.89   Cheese $6.59

Quesadilla
Melted jack cheese in a grilled flour tortilla with guacamole, sour cream & fresh pico de gallo on the side $4.89
Chicken, steak or pork quesadilla   add $1.89   Vegetarian style   add $1.29

SALAD

Bonita Tostada $5.45
Romaine in a large crisp tortilla shell, topped with black beans, tomato, cheese, guacamole, sour cream & homemade vinaigrette dressing.

With chicken, steak or pork   add $1.85

Bonita Ensalada $6.89
Marinated, chargrilled chicken tossed with crisp romaine lettuce, crispy tortilla strips, pico de gallo, olive oil vinaigrette dressing, tossed to order and topped with shaved cheese

Nachos $5.39
Tortilla chips covered with melted jack and cheddar cheese, black beans, sour cream, guacamole and fresh pico de gallo

Try it with chicken, pork or steak   add $1.19

TACOS
Warm flour tortillas, stuffed with jack cheese, diced tomatoes and lettuce.

Taco Meal
Any 3 of our tacos. Chicken, steak or pork. Served with a side of guacamole $5.89

Individual Taco
Charbroiled Steak	$2.65
Marinated Chicken	$2.65
Braised Pork	$2.65
Ground Beef	$2.65
Vegetarian	$2.50
(black beans, peppers & onions)

SIDE ORDERS
Chips		$1.89
Guacamole	**Small**	$1.89
Guacamole 8 oz side w/chips		$4.29
Fresh salsa made fresh daily 8 oz		$1.89
Rice or Beans (pinto or black)		$1.89
Sour Cream		$0.50

FAJITAS
Platter of charbroiled chicken, steak or pork grilled peppers, onions, rice, beans, sour cream and guacamole.
Corn or flour tortillas $7.95

Olde Tyme
Pub & Grill

≪ Appetizers ≫

Wings
Our Wings Served with Bleu Cheese & Celery
Served Buffalo, Honey Hot, Sesame Teriyaki $5.95

Super Nachos
Our Fresh Homemade Tortilla Chips Covered
with Melted Cheddar & Topped with
Homemade Chili, Black Olives, Onions,
Chopped Tomatoes, Jalapenos, Salsa,
Sour Cream, & Guacamole. $6.95

≪ Soups/Salads ≫

New England Clam Chowder
Our Homemade Classic Rich & Creamy Fresh
Maine Clams. Served to Your Liking:
                    Cup - $2.00   Bowl - $3.95

**Grilled Chicken or Grilled Shrimp over
Field Greens**
Fresh Breast Grilled & Seared Julienned Field
Greens with Ripe Tomato, Cucumber,
Onions, & Peppers.
          Chicken - $8.99   Or   Shrimp - $9.95

≪ Burgers/Sandwiches ≫

"Hot" Corned Beef
Homemade *on Rye with Mustard* $6.95

Burger Deluxe
Our 1/2 Pounder Grilled to Your Liking Served
with Fresh Cut Idaho Fries. $5.95

Two Fisted Burger Deluxe
Our Double Pounder Grilled to Your Liking
Served with Fresh Cut Idaho Fries. $7.95

Fried Catfish
Freshly Caught Catfish "Cajun" Herbed Served
on a Club Hero With Russian. $6.95

Quesadilla
Steak, Chicken, or Shrimp with Melted Jack &
Cheddar Cheese in a Flour Tortilla.
          Chicken/Steak - $6.95   Shrimp - $7.95

≪ Entrees ≫
All Entrees Served with Soup or Salad

Steak & Chops
Hand Trimmed Grilled 12oz New York Strip
with Baker/Mash & Vegetable $14.95
with Shrimp Scampi $17.95

Pan Fried Pork Chops with Sautéed Cherry
Peppers and Rosemary with Baker/Rice &
Vegetable. $13.95

Fish & Seafood
Pan Seared "Wild" Trout $12.95
Shrimp Scampi Served Over Linguini $14.95
Dijon Encrusted Salmon in Cream Sauce $13.95
Beer Battered Grouper & Chips $12.95

Chicken
Roasted 1/2 Chicken with Sage Stuffing $12.95
Chicken Vino Blanco with Eggplant $14.95
Chicken Marsala in Sautéed Mushrooms $13.95
Chicken Piccata with Lemon,
Capers, & Wine $13.95
Chicken Tiverina with Prosciutto
& Eggplant $15.95
Chicken Pot Pie *Old Fashioned Mash Crust* $12.95
Chicken Francese *Egg Dipped with Lemon* $13.95

Pasta
Pasta Primavera *Fresh Vegetables with Your Choice
of Creamy Alfredo or Our Homemade Marinara*
          $10.95
Penne A La Vodka *Shallot, Garlic, Vodka Flamed
With Prosciutto, Peas, & Penne* $12.95
Pasta Portafino *Penne, Chicken, Sausage,
Mushroom, Sundried Tomato in
Our Special Sauce* $14.95

≪ Kids Corner ≫

Burger with Fresh Idaho Fries $4.95
Grilled Cheese with Fresh Fries $4.95
Chicken Fingers with Fresh Fries $4.95
Chicken Breast with Fresh Fries $4.95

* PRICES ARE SUBJECT TO CHANGE WITHOUT NOTICE.

Olde Tyme Pub & Grill

≪ *Appetizers* ≫

Wings
Our Wings Served with Bleu Cheese & Celery
Served Buffalo, Honey Hot, Sesame Teriyaki $5.95

Super Nachos
Our Fresh Homemade Tortilla Chips Covered
with Melted Cheddar & Topped with
Homemade Chili, Black Olives, Onions,
Chopped Tomatoes, Jalapenos, Salsa,
Sour Cream, & Guacamole. $6.95

≪ *Soups/Salads* ≫

New England Clam Chowder
Our Homemade Classic Rich & Creamy Fresh
Maine Clams. Served to Your Liking:
Cup - $2.00   Bowl - $3.95

**Grilled Chicken or Grilled Shrimp over
Field Greens**
Fresh Breast Grilled & Seared Julienned Field
Greens with Ripe Tomato, Cucumber,
Onions, & Peppers.
Chicken - $8.99   Or   Shrimp - $9.95

≪ *Burgers/Sandwiches* ≫

"Hot" Corned Beef
Homemade *on Rye with Mustard* $6.95

Burger Deluxe
Our 1/2 Pounder Grilled to Your Liking Served
with Fresh Cut Idaho Fries. $5.95

Two Fisted Burger Deluxe
Our Double Pounder Grilled to Your Liking
Served with Fresh Cut Idaho Fries. $7.95

Fried Catfish
Freshly Caught Catfish "Cajun" Herbed Served
on a Club Hero With Russian. $6.95

Quesadilla
Steak, Chicken, or Shrimp with Melted Jack &
Cheddar Cheese in a Flour Tortilla.
Chicken/Steak - $6.95   Shrimp - $7.95

≪ *Entrees* ≫

All Entrees Served with Soup or Salad

Steak & Chops
Hand Trimmed Grilled 12oz New York Strip
with Baker/Mash & Vegetable $14.95
with Shrimp Scampi $17.95
Pan Fried Pork Chops with Sautéed Cherry
Peppers and Rosemary with Baker/Rice &
Vegetable $13.95

Fish & Seafood
Pan Seared "Wild" Trout $12.95
Shrimp Scampi Served Over Linguini $14.95
Dijon Encrusted Salmon in Cream Sauce $13.95
Beer Battered Grouper & Chips $12.95

Chicken
Roasted 1/2 Chicken with Sage Stuffing $12.95
Chicken Vino Blanco with Eggplant $14.95
Chicken Marsala in Sautéed Mushrooms $13.95
Chicken Piccata with Lemon,
Capers, & Wine $13.95
Chicken Tiverina with Prosciutto
& Eggplant $15.95
Chicken Pot Pie *Old Fashioned Mash Crust* $12.95
Chicken Francese *Egg Dipped with Lemon* $13.95

Pasta
Pasta Primavera *Fresh Vegetables with Your Choice
of Creamy Alfredo or Our Homemade Marinara*
$10.95
Penne A La Vodka *Shallot, Garlic, Vodka Flamed
With Prosciutto, Peas, & Penne* $12.95
Pasta Portafino *Penne, Chicken, Sausage,
Mushroom, Sundried Tomato in
Our Special Sauce* $14.95

≪ *Kids Corner* ≫

Burger with Fresh Idaho Fries	$4.95
Grilled Cheese with Fresh Fries	$4.95
Chicken Fingers with Fresh Fries	$4.95
Chicken Breast with Fresh Fries	$4.95

* PRICES ARE SUBJECT TO CHANGE WITHOUT NOTICE.

Monitoring and Blood Testing

O f all of the steps you take to living better and really taking control of your diabetes, none is more important or helpful than successfully and carefully monitoring your blood sugar levels. It kills me when patients come into my office and when I ask them what their blood sugar test has been showing, they don't know what I am talking about or, even worse, tell me that the doctor says it's fine.

What does that mean? How can you set goals for yourself, plan your life, and manage your diabetes unless you know what normal blood sugar levels are supposed to be, what your numbers are now, what they were before, and what makes them go up or down? Knowledge is a very powerful tool, but only if you really understand the why, when, how, and what of blood sugar monitoring. Therefore, let's work on getting you as much information on blood sugars as possible.

Here's a friendly bit of advice. Your friends and some well-meaning health professionals will sometimes give you blood sugar numbers that are incorrect, so always be sure that you keep informed of the latest in diabetes numbers. These days, diabetes is being managed much more aggressively than it was years ago, and the recommended blood sugar numbers have changed frequently over the last few years, so it's hard to keep up with all of this new information, much like with diabetes medications. These changes in blood sugar numbers have occurred because data now tell us that complications start happening at much lower blood sugar levels than we previously believed. If we want to prevent these dangerous complications, then we have to keep blood sugars under much tighter control. Scientific evidence has shown that among people who are newly diagnosed with type 2 diabetes, up to 50% of them already have one or more diabetes complications. This is because people usually don't go to the doctor until they have the symptoms of a complication, which, sadly, is already pretty far along in the disease process.

It is a good idea to always check several sources to make sure you have the most up-to-date information. I also have to check the numbers frequently because information is updated constantly and we really want to be aware of the state-of-the-art treatments in diabetes. You'll also feel more confident in the numbers you have been shown when you can see the same ones in several places. I suggest that you go to the American Diabetes Association's website and click on the All About Diabetes link or give them a call at 1-800-DIABETES. There you will find enough information to form a good basic understanding of how diabetes is diagnosed and what numbers you should remember.

Let's talk about the ins and outs of blood sugar monitoring and the different tests and what they mean. This will help you understand why we have changed those numbers so radically over the past few years.

BLOOD SUGAR NUMBERS AND YOU

Why are blood sugar numbers so important? First, they tell you the status of your diabetes right now. Your numbers show how much sugar (glucose) has been in your blood in the past three months and help guide us in deciding what plans should be made in your care. Your numbers allow us to set goals for you and help you and your health care team develop a treatment plan specifically for you. So, let's look at the blood glucose tests that may be ordered for you and discuss what each tells us about you.

Fasting Blood Sugar

Your fasting blood sugars tell you what your blood sugar level is when you have not eaten anything or had anything to drink in the previous eight hours. This test is usually done in the laboratory, but you can also do it yourself with a home glucose monitor in the morning before you have any-thing to eat or drink. When you have to come into the clinic for laboratory work, you will normally be told to be NPO, which is a fancy way of telling you to avoid eating or drink-ing anything prior to the test. (NPO is an acronym for the Latin phrase, *noti per os*, which means "nothing by mouth.")

Testing your fasting blood sugar level is important be-cause all of the planning involved in determining which med-ications or diabetes treatments to give you starts with know-ing two things: 1) what your blood sugar level is without food and 2) how your blood sugar responds to food or drink.

Normal fasting blood sugar levels fall between 70 and 99 mg/dl. This is the amount of sugar needed by your body to keep it functioning. When your blood sugar levels start to rise above this range, there are two categories of abnormal blood sugar levels. The first is called impaired glucose toler-ance, and it falls between 100 and 125 mg/dl. If your levels are more than 125 mg/dl, you'll be diagnosed with diabetes. I don't really bother with these specifics, because as far as I am concerned, once your levels rise above 100 mg/dl, you've got abnormal blood sugar levels. So let's not bicker about what's normal and what's impaired glucose tolerance

A Lesson in Numbers

Please understand that when I started writing this book, the normal blood sugar numbers were 70–110 mg/dl. In less than one year, the numbers have been revised because of new evidence in scientific research. Again, evidence has proven that the tighter you maintain blood sugar control, the less chance you have of developing diabetes complications. See? I'm continually learning and studying these numbers. You should be, too.

and diabetes, because once those average fasting levels creep higher and higher, something needs to be done. This is so important that I am going to repeat that last statement again: your blood sugar is either normal or not normal. There is no such thing as a little bit of sugar, high normal, almost diabetes, or my real favorite "borderline diabetes." Hearing this gives me chest pains. How can something be almost normal or almost abnormal?

What Is Pre-Diabetes?

Please do not equate what people call "borderline" with the term "pre-diabetes." Pre-diabetes means that your body is not adequately using your glucose and if intervention does not occur, you will develop diabetes. Before people develop type 2 diabetes, they almost always have "pre-diabetes." When you have pre-diabetes, your blood sugar levels are higher than normal, but not yet high enough to give a diagnosis of diabetes.

There are 41 million people in the U.S., aged 40–74, who have pre-diabetes. Recent research has shown that some long-term damage to the body, especially the heart and circulatory system, may already be occurring in people with pre-diabetes.

Research has also shown that if you take action to manage your blood sugar levels when you have pre-diabetes, you
can delay or even prevent type 2 diabetes from developing.

TIME FOR A BLOOD SUGAR TEST

If there is anything more important than knowing your
blood sugar numbers and how they connect to your health
and well-being, it is knowing when to test your blood sugars and recognizing the signs and symptoms of either high
or low blood sugars. You're probably already somewhat
familiar with the effects of high or low blood sugar on your
well-being. It is not fun feeling tired and heavy all of the
time. Neither is it fun feeling shaky and headachy either.
Can you imagine living every day of your entire life with
these feelings? This is not a great way to live your life.

I have pre-diabetes, and when my blood sugar is just a
little bit high, my vision gets blurry. This is a pain, but at
least because the effects are so obvious, I immediately
know when my blood sugar levels are high. But I don't rely
on these suspicions; I also test my blood to verify it.

This is a very important concept. You may think you
know when your blood sugar is high or low and decide that
you don't actually need to check your blood sugar levels.
That is not a good strategy. Sometimes blood sugar lows
and highs feel differently on different days, and it may be
difficult to decide what those feelings mean. Why would
you take a chance on treating the low blood sugar you think
you are having when you might actually have high blood
sugar? If you've misread your symptoms, you've just added
more glucose to a very high blood sugar level and can make
yourself very ill. You don't guess if your car has too much or
too little gas, you check the gas gauge. So why would you
guess about your blood sugar levels? Always test!

The Risks of Being Unaware

It has always been interesting to me that patients who have been walking around with very high blood sugars (above 200–250 mg/dl) tell me that they feel just fine. Then we get their blood sugars under control, and they tell me that they feel "strange" or "not too good." The person's body has adapted over time to this thick blood sugar, and they are not aware of how a healthy blood sugar level feels. This can be very difficult to explain and is somewhat upsetting to the person.

Do understand that it will not take long for you and your body to adapt and come to terms with this new way of living. You will feel less tired and have more energy. Believe me; you'll know right away when your blood sugars get closer and closer to normal levels. Better yet, you will reduce your risk of developing those nasty complications of diabetes.

Feeling Funny? Test!

How often should you be testing your blood? That depends on you, your health status, and what information your doctor or educator needs to help you maintain good blood sugar levels. People with type 1 diabetes may test as few as four times a day but usually test about seven times a day. People with type 2 diabetes often test four times a day but may test twice a day when their blood sugar levels are well managed. Some people who regularly have the same values at the same time on every day may only test their blood sugar levels twice a week. It takes a lot of work to get to that point, though.

I bet you're thinking something like this: "Okay Ginger, I get it, but how many times do I have to check my blood sugar?" Well, I'm not going to answer that! Every person is different, and you need to test when *you* need to test, not someone else. So set up that appointment with your doctor and diabetes educator.

I will tell you that the usual test times are first thing in the morning and before you eat anything. This reading will give you your fasting blood sugar, which tells us what your base blood sugar is without any food influencing the levels. We then test before each meal and before bedtime. This is the usual four times a day testing cycle that has been used for years. You will also likely be asked to take an additional test called the two-hour postprandial test. These tests are done two hours after you have eaten a meal and tell us how your body responds to meals. The target blood sugar level of this test is below 180 mg/dl.

Pattern Management

Remember, blood sugar testing puts you in control of your diabetes. It tells you what your blood sugar is at that precise moment. It will let you find out which foods raise your blood sugar a lot and which foods do not. It will tell you if your medications are working or if they need to be changed. Keeping a record of your blood tests and giving that information to your health care providers (so they have data to make accurate decisions about your treatment) is very proactive and a major part of the partnership you develop with the people who care for you and about you. When you keep a solid blood sugar log, you and your health care provider can work together to interpret the information. Then, the two of you can work together in forming goals, such as adjusting your meal plan, your medication, and your physical activity, to help you manage your diabetes.

This is called **pattern management**. I ask my patients to keep a blood glucose log. These logs tell me so much about a patient's diabetes and how his or her blood sugar levels respond to everything the patient does. You should be keep-

ing a logbook as well. Don't forget to bring your logbook
with you when you visit your doctor or diabetes educator.

Logbooks: Take Control!

Bud's Food and Sugar Diary

Date	Meal	Food description
1/3/06		
Weight 178 lbs	Breakfast	Eggs (2) Mushrooms Onion (1/4 cup) Cheese (2 slices) Water (10 oz) Olive oil (1 Tbsp)
Physical activity Walked 3 miles before lunch, after test	Snack	Peanuts (20) Diet Coke (12 oz)
	Lunch	Chicken noodle soup Salad (w/o dressing) Dressing, balsamic (2 Tbsp) Pineapple (1/4 cup) Cottage cheese (1/4 cup) Diet Coke (16 oz)
	Snack	Peanuts (20) Diet Coke (12 oz)
	Dinner	Chicken noodle soup Pineapple (1/2 cup) Water (10 oz)
	Snack	Tostadas (4) w/ salsa
	Total	

This is a copy of a record kept by one of my patients who is committed to lowering his blood sugars and is trying to avoid starting medications. Two weeks after we discussed tactics to achieve his goals, he lost eight pounds and

Calories	Carb grams	Fat grams	Fiber grams	Protein grams	Sugar level
150	2	9	—	10	119
9	3.5	—	0.5	1	
23	5.3	—	0.8	0.8	
70	2	4	—	3	
—	—	—	—	—	
120	—	14	—	—	
40	1	4	0.5	2	
—	—	—	—	—	
75	9	2	1	4	
132	28.5	—	9.5	7.5	
50	3	5	—	—	
19	4.75	0.25	0.5	0.25	
40	3	1	—	13	
—	—	—	—	—	
40	1	4	0.5	2	
—	—	—	—	—	
75	9	2	1	4	
38	9.5	0.5	1	0.5	
—	—	—	—	—	
50	7	2	—	—	
931	88.55	47.75	15.3	48.05	

(continued)

Bud's Food and Sugar Diary (Continued)

Date	Meal	Food description
1/4/06		
Weight 178 lbs	Breakfast	Eggs (2) Morningstar sausage patty Olive oil (1 Tbsp) Water (10 oz)
	Snack	Diet Coke (8 oz)
Physical activity Walked 3 miles after test, before lunch	Lunch	Egg drop soup (1 cup) String beans (1/4 cup) Onions and peppers (1/4 cup) Mushrooms (1/2 cup) Fried rice (1/2 cup) Chicken, dark (4 oz) Hot tea (8 oz) Water (18 oz)
	Snack	Nuts Diet Coke (12 oz) Water (10 oz)
	Dinner	Salmon (4 oz) Broccoli (1 cup) Asparagus (8 spears) Cheese (1 slice) Pineapple (1/2 cup)
	Total	

developed an understanding of which foods make a difference in his blood sugar management.

Bud, my patient, developed this chart. He used this chart to compile the information I needed to do pattern management. I now know what his fasting blood sugar is every morning and how specific foods change his blood

Calories	Carb grams	Fat grams	Fiber grams	Protein grams	Sugar level
150	2	10	—	10	140
80	3	3	—	10	
120	—	14	—	—	
—	—	—	—	—	
—	—	—	—	—	
205	3	3	—	5	141
22	5	—	—	—	
40	8	—	—	—	
30	4	—	—	—	
126	29	2	—	—	
200	1	15	—	—	
—	—	—	—	—	
—	—	—	—	—	
40	1	3	—	2	174
—	—	—	—	—	
—	—	—	—	—	
248	—	12	—	32	
25	5	—	3	3	
28	6	—	2	4	
35	1	2	—	2	
50	30	—	—	—	
1399	98	64	5	58	123

sugar. I can counsel him on his meal plan and assess his need for medications.

When I look at the table it tells me several things. I know what Bud's blood sugar is in the morning and two hours after each meal. I know how much Bud eats at his meals and which foods make his blood sugar go up a little and which foods make it go up drastically. I told him that he was not eating enough on several days and that I did not want him to be hungry because it would make him frustrated and affect his management.

Before you get frightened by the number of blood tests on this log please be aware that he kept this record for several days, so I had enough information to set goals with him. We had agreed that he would lose five pounds over two months, but he lost eight pounds in two weeks. This may surprise you, but I told him to slow down because losing too much weight too quickly would make it more difficult to predict and manage his blood sugar levels.

Take a look at Bud's logbook. Do you see the patterns I've been discussing? Do you see that Chinese food makes his blood sugar go up the highest? Chinese food is often cooked with a lot of sugar, so it can greatly affect blood sugar levels. I reminded Bud that Chinese vegetables are a better choice than Chinese honey-coated chicken.

Look at the foods on the list. If you were Bud's dietitian, would you be happy with Bud's meal plan? Are you surprised that some foods, such as a salad, make his blood sugar go higher than a hamburger? What is in the salad? If you put in noodles and oranges and regular salad dressing, you might as well eat a piece of cake. Those little add-ons can really pack a punch.

Taking Action

Pattern management allows you and your health care team to work together in assessing your current health status and set goals for the future. We might decide that you need to lose five pounds over the next two months. We might decide to set a goal for carbohydrates in your meal plan if we find that you eat too many carbohydrates before lunch, which is why your blood sugars are high before dinner. Or we could decide that pasta affects your blood sugars very quickly, so our goal would be to cut down on pasta to one serving a week.

But we can't set any of these goals if we don't know where we are now. Pattern management is like setting up an itinerary for a trip. I wouldn't ask for directions to Kentucky without telling someone where I'm starting from first. We would also check the map as we go to make sure that we are still headed in the right direction. Not many people with dia-

Pattern Management in Germany

Several years ago I was in Germany visiting a diabetes clinic and observing how that country takes care of people with diabetes. It was very interesting. All patients who are diagnosed are allowed to attend and live in a diabetes clinic for 12 days for free. It is run by teams comprised of a doctor, dietitian, certified diabetes educator, nurse, social worker or psychologist, pharmacist, and physical therapist. Impressive, isn't it?

Patients stay in this hostel and go to class every day. They are taught an intensive program and learn to care for themselves and their diabetes. They learn all about pattern management and even how to adjust their medications and insulin levels. (We teach many of our patients in the U.S. the same thing.)

When these people go home they are expected to guide their doctors in their care and to make sure that they are taking care of themselves and that their health care providers are making informed decisions about their care. Many of these trained patients return to small villages or towns in Germany, where the government is not always able to provide endocrinologists. This preventive strategy protects the health of German citizens. Isn't this an interesting idea? I think it would be great if we could do something like that in this country. Maybe we will someday.

betes seem to hear of pattern management, but it's one of the key tools in getting on track to better living with diabetes.

THE TOOLS OF BLOOD SUGAR MONITORING

So now you know why you check your blood sugar, and you should have a pretty good idea of when to check it. Are you ready for the big question? How do you check your blood sugar? I'll give you some tips on this here.

Let me tell you how simple it is to test your blood using today's modern technology. Using any of the new, simple lancing devices, you stick your finger to obtain a drop of blood. These lancing devices are very easy to use, and the needles are so small and thin that it's virtually painless. Because the amount of blood needed for the test is so small, you don't have to puncture deeply. Your blood is drawn into your monitor or dropped on a test strip, and the meter gives you the results in a short amount of time.

I'm going to talk to you about all of the tools that you, as a person with diabetes, and health care providers, as people who care for and about you, will use to monitor your blood sugars. They are fingersticking, lancing devices, blood glucose meters, urine tests, A1C tests, and oral glucose tolerance tests.

Fingersticking

Whenever you need to test your blood, you'll have to stick your finger, what we often call **fingersticking**. This is when you make a small pinprick in your fingertip and squeeze out a drop of blood, which is then measured by a blood glucose monitor. You're probably already doing this, so there's not too much more I need to say about it. However, I would like to give you some expert tips on fingersticks.

First, make sure you hold your hand below the level of your heart, doing this will allow the blood to flow down your arm and quickly out of the puncture. Don't raise your hand up in the air and expect to get blood easily from your fingertips. Doesn't that make sense? If your hands are up high, then the blood will flow away from your fingertips.

Second, take a look at your fingers, palm up. The centers of your fingers are very sensitive and have lots of nerve endings. The area around the edges is less sensitive, and it will be less painful to stick yourself there. Use those areas, and rotate the fingers frequently. Make sure you apply cream to your hands often and keep the skin clean and soft.

Third, carefully choose your hand cleansers. For many years we had people clean their fingers with alcohol before sticking themselves. This caused the skin to dry and sometimes crack, and it is no longer recommended unless you are in a place where you cannot wash your hands or the location is really not clean. Public bathrooms concern me because people are not always as clean and sanitary as they should be. Many health care providers recommend carrying one of those self-drying hand sanitizers, but try to find one that does not dry your skin. If you use alcohol to clean before fingersticking, plan on using moisturizing hand cream on a regular basis. Make sure you rub the hand cream in well, so you are not testing the sugar content of the cream instead of your blood.

Fourth, if you have trouble obtaining blood from a callused finger, you might want to soak your finger in warm water for a few minutes. Another technique you can use is to squeeze your finger with your thumb until the tip is red and filled with blood. Keep squeezing it while you lance the skin. This is one of my favorite methods, and when I use it, fingersticking hurts less and always provides enough blood. I've been demonstrating blood testing for so many years that you can believe me when I tell you how simple and painless this test can be.

Lancing Devices

Name (manufacturer/distributor)	Features and supplies
Accu-Chek Multiclix Lancet Device (Roche Diagnostics)	Eleven depth settings provide precise control of penetration depth to help avoid contact with nerves. Linear track design minimizes painful side-to-side motion. Uses the Accu-Chek Multiclix lancet drum of six preloaded lancets. Includes clear cap for alternate site testing. Includes two drums (12 lancets).
Accu-Chek Multiclix Lancet Drums (Roche Diagnostics)	For use with the Accu-Chek Multiclix lancet device. Drum of six preloaded lancets. Lancets are self-contained for enhanced safety. 30G lancets. Comes in packages of 102 and 204 (17 and 34 drums).
Accu-Chek Softclix Lancet Device (Roche Diagnostics)	Eleven depth settings provide precise control of penetration depth to help avoid contact with nerves. Linear track design minimizes painful side-to-side motion. Uses Accu-Chek Softclix lancets. Includes clear cap for alternate site testing. Includes 25 lancets.
Accu-Chek Softclix Lancets (Roche Diagnostics)	For use with the Accu-Chek Softclix and Accu-Chek Softclix Plus lancet devices. Comes in packages of 100 and 200. Tips are silicon coated.
Accu-Chek Soft Touch Lancet Device (Roche Diagnostics)	Five depth settings with an adjustable dial provide a personalized level of skin comfort while obtaining an adequate blood sample.
Accu-Chek Soft Touch Lancets (Roche Diagnostics)	Fits most lancet devices. Comes in packages of 100 and 200.
Aimsco Adjustable Lancet Device (Aimsco Delta Hi-Tech)	Five depth settings for greater comfort. Use with Aimsco Lancets.

Name (manufacturer/distributor)	Features and supplies
Aimsco Lancets (Aimsco Delta Hi-Tech)	28G and 30G. Compatible with most lancet devices.
Ames Gluco System Lancets (Bayer HealthCare, LLC, Diabetes Care Division)	Can be used in either Autolet or Glucolet.
Ascensia Microlet Adjustable Lancing Device (Bayer HealthCare, LLC, Diabetes Care Division)	Ergonomic design has easy cocking mechanism and five adjustable settings to control depth of puncture. A clear end cap is also provided for multiple site testing.
Ascensia Microlet Lancets (Bayer HealthCare, LLC, Diabetes Care Division)	For use with Ascensia Microlet Automatic Lancing Device and Ascensia Microlet Vaculance Lancing Device; 28G.
Ascensia Microlet Vaculance Lancing Device (Bayer HealthCare, LLC, Diabetes Care Division)	Vacuum action draws blood to skin surface, allowing patient to choose lancing sites less painful than fingertips, such as forearm, palm, abdomen, or thigh. Four lancing depths. Uses Ascensia Microlet lancets.
Auto-Lancet (Palco Labs, Inc.)	Adjustable-tip, reusable lancing device. Five depth settings, linear tracking, and quality design for maximum comfort and least capillary damage. Standard size. Fits most lancets. Two lancets included. Lifetime warranty.
Auto-Lancet Custom (Palco Labs, Inc.)	New design includes custom color and logo and an optional elastomer barrel for improved grip. Fits most lancets. Improved action in a sleek size, with a lifetime warranty.
Auto-Lancet Mini (Palco Labs, Inc.)	Same quality, features, and design as the Auto-Lancet, except in compact, mini size. Adjustable tip with 5 settings. Two lancets included. Lifetime warranty.

From the *Diabetes Forecast Resource Guide* (January 2007).

Take a look at the list of lancing devices on pages 126–127. As you can see, it also details the benefits of each and every model. Lancing devices are included in the kits that arrive with your blood glucose meter. The needles are so small that you rarely feel the stick at all, but there are some differences between the different models. You always have the alternative of buying a separate one that has features that you prefer. Some devices look like a long, thin pen. Some are attached to the meter, so you aren't carrying a separate item that you could lose or misplace. Are you always losing things? Consider a meter with an attached lancing device.

If you have more questions about choosing a device, talk to your health care provider. In many cases, you can even ask your pharmacist. Patients often talk to their pharmacists about their experiences with lancing devices, so he or she may be a valuable resource.

Please know that these lancing devices are different from the single-use ones you find in laboratories. Those are usually much more painful because they are bigger than the ones that you will use with your meter. Often, laboratories require more blood for their tests, so they have to use a larger lancet than you will for home use.

Blood Glucose Meters

You know how to get your blood now, but what do you do with it? Well, most likely, you're going to be using a blood glucose meter at home to check your blood sugar levels. A blood glucose meter is a small computer that reads your blood sugar sample. There is usually a short countdown on the screen and then your blood sugar levels pops up, just like on a calculator. Yes, it's really that simple.

If your doctor or diabetes educator decides that you can benefit from checking your blood sugar at home, then he or she will recommend that you get one of these monitors.

Often, the choice of specific meter is left to the diabetes educator or health professional who teaches you how to use it. However, if you feel ready for a meter and think that you'd like to check your levels at home, it can't hurt to ask your health care providers what they think of you getting one. Remember what I said way back in the beginning of this book? You're still the captain of your ship; don't forget that.

Choosing a Meter

There are many meters to choose from, and the meter you choose should be able to give you the information you want to know and suit your own personal needs. There are even meters that talk to you if you don't see well. Some meters only record the results from one test; others can

Here are some questions to think about while looking at a meter to buy.

- What meter does your doctor or diabetes educator suggest? He or she may have a particular meter that they use often and know best.
- What will it cost? Some insurance companies will only pay for a certain meter. Call your insurance company before you purchase a meter and ask how to get a meter and supplies. If your insurance company does not pay for blood glucose checking supplies, rebates are often available toward the purchase of your meter. You will still have to consider the cost of the matching strips and lancets. Shop around.
- How easy is the meter to use? Methods vary. Some have fewer steps than others.
- How simple is the meter to maintain? Is it easy to clean? How is the meter calibrated (set correctly for the batch of strips you are using)?

Name (manufacturer/ distributor)	Size (inches)	Weight (ounces)	Test strip used	Range (mg/dl)	Test time	Battery
Accu-Chek Active (Roche Diagnostics)	4.6 × 1.07 × 0.9	2.01 without batteries	Accu-Chek Active	10–600	5 sec.	(1) 3-volt
Accu-Chek Advantage (Roche Diagnostics)	3.3 × 2.8 × 0.8	1.8 without batteries	Accu-Chek Comfort Curve	10–600	26 sec.	(1) 3-volt coin cell #2032
Accu-Chek Aviva (Roche Diagnostics)	3.7 × 2.0 × 0.86	2.11 with battery	Accu-Chek Aviva	10–600	5 sec.	(1) 3-volt
Accu-Chek Compact Plus (Roche Diagnostics)	4.4 × 1.9 × 1.2 (without lancet device)	4.2 with batteries and test drum (without lancet device)	Accu-Chek Compact	10–600	5 sec.	(2) AAA
Accu-Chek Voicemate (Roche Diagnostics)	6.5 × 3.0 × 2.4	10.94 without batteries	Accu-Chek Comfort Curve	10–600	26 sec.	9-volt for the voice synthesizer (2) 3-volt in meter
Advance Intuition (Arkray)	3.9 × 2.3 × 0.8	2.2	Advance Intuition	30–550	10 sec.	3-volt (CR 2032)

Warranty	How calibrated	Control solution	Features
years	Snap-in code key	Yes	Two-step procedure. Monitor turns on automatically when strip is inserted. Alternate site testing; results are downloadable; small sample size; 7- and 14-day averaging. Rubber grips. English and Spanish instructions including a "First Time Guide." Toll-free call center 24 hours a day, 7 days a week, with multilingual reps.
years	Snap-in code key	Yes	Uses small sample size, capillary action, and large target area for easy dosing. Results are downloadable; 480-value memory with time and date; 7-, 14-, and 30-day averaging. Rubber grips. English and Spanish instructions including a "First Time Guide." Toll-free call center 24 hours a day, 7 days a week, with multilingual reps.
years	Snap-in code key	Yes	Wide-mouth dosing area attracts and holds blood sample allowing patients to fill the strip easily. Large, wide strip and rubber monitor grips provide easy handling. Alternate site testing; results are downloadable; 500-value memory with time and date; 0.6-microliter sample size; 7-, 14-, and 30-day averaging. English and Spanish instructions including a "First Time Guide." Toll-free call center 24 hours a day, 7 days a week, with multilingual reps.
years	No coding required	Yes	Detachable Accu-Chek Softclix Plus lancet device and no strip handling. Underdosed strip detection. Alternate site testing; results are downloadable; 300-value memory with time and date; 1.5-microliter sample size; 7-, 14-, and 30-day averaging. English and Spanish instructions including a "First Time Guide." Toll-free call center 24 hours a day, 7 days a week, with multilingual reps.
years	Snap-in code key	Yes	For the blind and visually impaired. Step-by-step voice guide. Touchable strips. Portable. No cleaning required. Lilly brand insulin identification ensures customer of correct insulin formulation. English and Spanish instructions including a "First Time Guide." Toll-free call center with multilingual reps.
years	Code chip	Yes	Two-step testing. Automatic on/off with strip insertion. 3-microliter sample size. One-button memory recall. Stores up to 10 tests. Large display screen. Guide-Me-Curve strips guide the finger to application site where blood is wicked onto test strip. 10-second test time.

(continued)

Name (manufacturer/ distributor)	Size (inches)	Weight (ounces)	Test strip used	Range (mg/dl)	Test time	Battery
Advance Micro-draw (Arkray)	3.0 × 2.5 × 0.5	1.5	Advance Micro-draw	20–600	15 sec.	3-volt (CR 2032)
AgaMatrix Wave 1 (AgaMatrix Inc.)	2.8 × 1.6 × 0.6	1.56	Liberty	20–600	Variable; 3–4 sec.	(2) 3-volt lithium
Ascensia Breeze Blood Glucose Monitoring System (Bayer HealthCare, LLC, Diabetes Care Division)	2.5 × 4.1 × 1.0	3.8	Ascensia Autodisc; 10 test strips in one disc	10–600	30 sec.	(1) 3-volt lithium

From the *Diabetes Forecast Resource Guide* (January 2007).

store the results from your last 50, 100, or 200 tests. Some meters are so fancy that they can keep all kinds of information, including what you eat and when you took your medications. Some meters allow you to download this information to a computer. Come to think of it, maybe blood glucose meters will someday put me out of a job!

You and your health care provider should select the right meter for you. It can be as simple or as sophisticated as you want it to be. This is an important decision. There are so many meters that choosing one can be exciting, too.

Definitely be aware that your insurance plan may be the deciding issue in which meter you wind up using. You should find out which meters your insurance will allow

/arranty	How calibrated	Control solution	Features
years	Code chip	Yes	Test strips wick the blood onto the end of the strip. 1.5-microliter sample size. Digital display, 250-test memory with time and date stamp. 14- and 30-day average and downloading capabilities with GlucoBalance data management software. Finger or palm testing.
/A	Code	Yes, 2 levels	WaveSense glucose monitoring technology makes monitor highly accurate. Variable test time; 3–4 seconds; less painful testing with 0.5-microliter sample (see blood enter strip). Large rubber grips. Monitor activates automatically after strip insertion. Mealtime and 14-, 30-, and 90-day averages/graphs on large, backlit display. Six alarms, including hypo/hyperglycemic alerts.
years	Automatic	Yes	Disc-based monitor; no coding. Underfill detection. Each function button does only one thing. Eliminates individual strip handling and performs 10 tests without reloading. Test strip automatically draws the amount of blood required. Downloadable memory for PC tracking. Stores up to 100 results. Alternate site testing. No cleaning necessary.

before you attend a training session with an educator. It makes no sense to have someone teach you how to use one meter and then find out that a different one is the only type you'll be able to afford.

The cost of meters is a real issue, and although Medicare, Medicaid, and most insurance companies are willing to pay for the meters and the strips, some coverage is very limited and can be an obstacle to strong blood sugar management. If your health care provider decides that you have to test more often than your plan allows, they can often get your plan to pay for more if the doctor writes a letter explaining your situation. Your partnership with your health care provider really makes a difference in this situation.

I recently had a meeting with a union delegate who was very upset that his union paid for strips but not for meters. I told him how to obtain meters for his members for little or no cost. Something can usually be arranged (see chapter 7). Regardless of how you get a meter, make sure that you get proper instruction. I've heard of people being handed their meter and told to read the instruction book. How is that helpful? You need to have an actual demonstration of a meter's operation and be able show the person that you can test your blood sugar correctly. Some meters require coding, cleaning, and priming, and all of those things need to be thoroughly explained.

The table on pages 130–133 describes many new meters and how much blood they require as well as the length of time needed for testing. All of the companies that man-

Why Should I Trust This Thing?

Experts have tested these meters in their labs and found them to be accurate and precise. That's the good news. The bad news is that meter mistakes most often come from the person doing the blood checks. For good results you need to do each step correctly. Here are other things that can cause your meter to give a poor reading.

- a dirty meter
- a meter or strip that's not at room temperature
- an outdated test strip
- a meter not set up for the current box of test strips
- a blood drop that is too small

Ask your health care team to check your skills at least once a year. Error can creep in over time.

ufacture these meters also produce wonderful education materials, but this is a complete list for you to check out and see what might be perfect for you. When you attend a diabetes self-management education program the educator will show you several meters, discuss the features and benefits of each, and help you decide which one will be best for you.

Many blood glucose meters allow you to do alternative site testing. That means you can draw blood from your palm or your forearm instead of your fingertips, which may be more sensitive. This is a great feature of many new meters. In the past, blood glucose meters needed a lot of blood to conduct a blood sugar test. Now, with improved technology, you don't need as much blood for testing, so you can draw it from other, less painful sites.

Using Your Meter to Manage Diabetes

Are you tired of keeping logs by now? Well, you're not done yet. An especially important component of blood sugar monitoring is keeping the records of your tests and linking the information to your activities. These can be kept in a log that is included with your meter and is given out freely by most meter and strip companies. At every health fair I have ever attended, someone is giving out glucose logs. Make sure that you get one. If you'd rather make your own, there's a sample one on page 136.

Many companies on the list also have software programs that allow you to manage your information on your computer. Check the list of meters, and they will tell you which companies allow this handy feature. This is wonderful because it allows you to e-mail that data to your health care providers if you have a problem or just want to show off your good blood sugar management. This is a lot of fun.

Week of _____

	Breakfast	Lunch	Dinner	Snack	Bedtime
Monday TIME					
Tuesday TIME					
Wednesday TIME					
Thursday TIME					
Friday TIME					
Saturday TIME					
Sunday TIME					

From the *American Diabetes Association Blood Glucose Log Book.*

Some insulin pumps, the Guardian RT Continuous Glucose Monitoring System by Medtronic, for example, allow you to continuously monitor your blood sugar levels and give you a complete picture of how your body adapts to the foods you eat, the exercise you do, and the medications you take. Can you imagine? You don't have to test to get a brief snapshot of your blood sugar levels; instead you get a com-plete profile of your blood sugar levels over an extended amount of time. These devices also have alerts that tell you when your blood sugar is going up or down. This is especially important for people who have hypoglycemia unawareness, which means that they do not recognize or feel the symptoms that indicate that their blood sugar is dangerously low. These are amazing little machines, but they are also really new.

Urine Testing

Until the 1980s, there was no such thing as a home blood glucose monitor and the only way to measure your blood sugar was by testing your urine. We now know that many patients can have high levels of blood sugar before they "spill sugar" into their urine. Relying on sugar in your urine to evaluate your overall blood sugar levels is risky because kidney function and too many other variables factor into the test results to be considered acceptable at this stage of diabetes care. From urine tests, we can only tell if you have no sugar or a small, medium, or large amount of sugar in your urine. That's fine, but we're really interesting in how much sugar is in *your blood*. Still, you may hear that there are still people who regularly test their urine, but there are usually only two circumstances where this is necessary.

One such situation occurs when a patient is somehow unable to acquire or pay for blood glucose testing equipment or maintain a regular supply of strips. This is a terrible situation. Any health care provider can usually find a way to acquire a meter and, at least, a small supply of strips to allow someone to monitor his or her blood sugar instead of through urine testing, which tends to be inaccurate. I would certainly prefer that you test your blood less often than rely on inaccurate urine testing.

The other situation when urine testing is used arises when a person absolutely refuses to test his or her blood for religious or phobic reasons. Cultural issues come with the territory when you deal with people, and if a health care provider cannot respect your personal reasons for not testing your blood, then he or she should not be teaching or caring for people with diabetes or any other condition.

There is one routine urine test that is important and should be considered by anyone with diabetes: testing for ketones in the urine. Ketones show up in your urine if your body is burning fat instead of glucose, which is a sign that things are not working so well. When the body is unable to burn glucose for energy (because there is not enough insulin to carry glucose into the cells or the body is resistant to its own insulin), it will burn what it

If you are required to test your urine, here's how the procedure normally goes.

- Get a sample of your urine in a clean container.
- Place the strip in the sample (you can also pass the strip through the urine stream).
- Gently shake excess urine off the strip.
- Wait for the strip pad to change color. The directions will tell you how long to wait.
- Compare the strip pad to the color chart on the strip bottle. This gives you a range of the amount of ketones in your urine.
- Record your results.

can to survive, which means that the body begins to burn its fat stores for energy. Ketones are a byproduct of this process, and they are poisonous to the body. This condition is called diabetic ketoacidosis and is discussed in detail in chapter 8.

Laboratory Tests

Two other lab tests give us a better view of a person's diabetes status. One in particular has changed the way we set and measure blood sugar goals.

A1C Test

Let's talk about A1C tests. This is a lab test. You may have also heard it called a hemoglobin A1C or glycosylated hemoglobin test. We now just call it an A1C test because it's easier to say.

An A1C test shows what your blood sugars have been averaging over the previous three months. It is shown as a percentage. Normal A1C levels are usually 4–6% in most labs. The American Diabetes Association recommends that A1C levels be kept below 7% for people with diabetes. On an individual basis, the ADA recommends keeping A1C levels as close to 6% as possible while avoiding very low blood sugar (hypoglycemic) episodes.

It is recommended that people with well managed blood sugar levels have an A1C test at least twice a year and that people with less stable blood sugar levels have an A1C test four times a year. This important test is a requirement of good diabetes care, so be sure you're having it done. If not, then be sure to ask your health care providers to give you one.

Many people with diabetes are diagnosed with very high A1C levels. High blood sugar levels lead to complications over time, and we know that lowering your blood sugar can greatly decrease your chances of developing complications. A1C is important because it offers a stable picture of your overall blood sugar levels. Your daily checks can fluctuate with food intake, exercise, and other variables, so they do not give your health care providers the "big picture" like A1C does. If your A1C levels are consistently high, then you run a higher risk of developing complications. I shouldn't have to say this, but you really need to work to keep your A1C level down.

Oral Glucose Tolerance Test (OGTT)
Although the fasting plasma glucose test is the preferred test to diagnose diabetes in children and adults who are not pregnant, some physicians prefer to do the oral glucose tolerance test. This is also a lab test and requires the person to have blood and urine tested while fasting (meaning that you have not eaten or drunk anything in the past eight hours). The patient is then given a drink high in glucose and tested again several times over the next two hours. This test is expensive, takes a long time, and is sometimes uncomfortable for the patients, so it is not done too often. When it is requested it is often because the health care provider is having a tough time deciding whether a person has type 1 or type 2 diabetes and wants to be sure before planning future care. This is very important because the treatments are very different for each disease.

There was a time not too long ago when we decided that only children got juvenile diabetes or insulin-dependent diabetes mellitus, which we now call type 1 diabetes. If you were an adult, then you had non–insulin-dependent diabetes mellitus or adult-onset diabetes, which we now call type 2 diabetes. This process was fundamentally wrong because different people can get different types of diabetes and getting the wrong treatment for a certain kind of diabetes didn't lead to a healthy, happy lifestyle. Thank goodness that we've learned about the differences between these two diseases and how to treat them.

Five

Movement

L et's talk about moving. Most people and books call it
"exercise," but I hate that word. Instead, I like to call it
something fun and easy, like "increasing your activity level"
or "motion." "Exercise" makes me think of gyms, stretch
pants, sweat, pain, and all of the things that go with that
image. It's never turned me on! Even though I know how
important moving is, whenever the word "exercise" gets
into my head, I get uncomfortable. Isn't that a terrible thing
for a diabetes educator to say? But just because I say this
doesn't mean that I'm not committed to the health benefits
that you'll get from increasing your activity level, and it certainly doesn't mean that I think we should just sit around
all the time. At the same time, however, just because I don't
like the gym doesn't mean that you can't like it either. So, if
you already go and really enjoy getting your motion there,
then you keep on doing it. Actually, I may kind of envy you
for that.

For those of us who aren't fans of exercise, we need to
find something less intimidating and overwhelming. Think
about what you like to do for fun and about what gets your
body moving. For example, I have always been a person
who loves the water, and for six months of the year, I live
in the Florida Keys. I always enjoyed swimming, but last

year I really got into water aerobics and discovered that it was not only fun but made a big impact on my life. I was going to class two mornings a week and discovered that I felt so much better after class that I started doing it on my own every morning. I even got to the point where I was swimming in the cold January and February months, so I bought a wet suit to keep warm. I bet I lost a couple of pounds just getting in and out of that tight thing. After a few weeks I noticed that my energy level was up and my blood pressure was down. My back, which had literally been a pain for years, felt much better. When I did not have the time to get some motion in my day, then I found myself really missing it.

An Inspiring Person

I know this wonderful lady, Coralie, who attends my water aerobics class. She's in her eighties and is fairly frail. Coralie always arrives in a wheelchair, but this charming woman is determined to do the best she can to survive her disabilities. She lives on a boat on our dock, and her husband wheels her over to the pool. No matter how chilly it is (and a wet suit is too difficult for her to put on), she eases herself into the water and does her exercises every single day. Sometimes she is the only one in the pool because the tourists think it's a little too cold. When I think about avoiding the water I just look at Coralie and get in.

"Coralie," I always say, "isn't it a bit cold in that water?"

"Ginger," she responds, "I've got plenty of years ahead of me when I won't feel hot or cold, so while I'm here, I'm going to do my best to keep going. Don't you have some exercises you're supposed to do?"

If that does not inspire you to get up and get going, nothing will.

GET YOURSELF IN MOTION

You can make motion a part of your daily life in so many ways. A lot of times, the first place to start is to think about what you do every day and what you like to do for fun. I do have one rule for you, though; don't tell me that you like to watch TV or surf the Internet. That's not motion, unless you count hand and eye motions, but you're not going to get into shape doing that. Let me give you an example from my life.

I love to dance, so I go out as often as I can. My husband and I belong to a square dance club, and we go every Tuesday night. There are usually four squares—that's 36 people—and we dance for two and a half hours. Most of the people are in their seventies and eighties, so I am usually the youngest person. No kidding! Studies have shown that people cover almost five to seven miles during an evening of square dancing. I bet you thought exercise had to be work and couldn't be fun. My friend Charles is eighty-six years old and a retired dentist. He is a wonderful dancer and the fastest jitterbugger I ever saw. His footwork is so incredible that I can barely keep up with him. I know I get an aerobic workout after one session of "Leroy Brown."

The other real issue is weight control. No one debates or doubts that if you want to lose weight there are two ways. One, you eat less, and two, you start moving. That's all there is to it. Like most Americans I spend a lot of time working in front of my computer, sitting on planes and in meetings, and not doing all the things the early people did. We no longer have to forage for food or outrun predators so we spend a lot of time sitting around.

Very few of us bother walking anywhere anymore so the most movement we make is getting in and out of the car to go someplace. Too often it is to the store to buy food or the restaurant to eat it. You need to take an inventory of the amount of movement you make every day and take a hard look at your lifestyle.

MOVING IS GOOD FOR YOU

Let's talk about what happens to your body when you start moving. If you have type 2 diabetes, then your health care providers may have discussed exercise with you but not gone over the many clinical benefits that it provides. Let's do that now.

Improved Sense of Well-Being

Here is an important thing to remember: exercise improves your sense of well-being. When you exercise, you'll feel proud of yourself as you see yourself achieving your goals. When you move more, you start to lose weight, and everything that was falling down on your body seems to lift up or at least feel like it is lifting up. You'll also feel an added burst of energy in your days or maybe a little more bounce in your step. Because you're doing something good *for* yourself, you begin to feel good *about* yourself. Want to know a secret? Try getting your friends and family to get into motion with you. If they're helping you out with your diabetes, then you can help them out a little with some exercise. Everyone wins when they bring motion into their lives.

Reduced Risk of Heart Disease

You can keep your heart healthy and working properly by giving it some work. By work, I mean that you should increase your heart rate on a regular basis. Doing this will improve your blood pressure, lower your bad cholesterol, and raise your good cholesterol.

Weight Loss

It's time for a learning activity. Don't worry; it only takes
15 minutes and a few props. Pick up three items: a two-
pound bag of flour or sugar, a five-pound bag, and a
10-pound bag. First, stand for five minutes and hold the
10-pound bag in front of your tummy. Just stand there and
hold the bag. Get someone else to time you. Then, grab the
five-pound bag and hold it on your back while leaning
over. Do this for five minutes as well. Tired yet? We're
almost done. Next, hold the two-pound bag in your hands,
holding your arms out in front of your body for another
five minutes. See how you feel when you finally put the
bags down, and you will be amazed. After that, think about
walking around with those weights all over you day in and
day out, because that's what you're carrying around all the
time if you're just 17 pounds overweight. Now, really think
about how you felt when you put the bags down. It felt
pretty good, didn't it?

After you learn something about carrying this weight,
try it with a few of your friends or family. You don't have
to lose a ton a weight to feel its effects. As you can see (and
probably feel right now) losing just 17 pounds can make a
world of difference.

If you walk one mile a day for three days a week, you
can lose half a pound a week. Now before you tell me that
half a pound is nothing, think about it this way: you're
looking at losing 26 pounds in one year. Would you be
happy to lose 26 pounds? Of course you would! I hear
patients complain that their doctors have told them that
they should lose 50 pounds and they are overwhelmed and
upset because it sounds impossible. It sounds awful to me
as well, because when I try to do something and don't succeed, I can get depressed or want to give up. Does that
sound familiar? Of course it does.

What if I asked you if you could lose five pounds over the next two months? Do you think you could do that? Is this a realistic goal? If you are starting to tell me all the reasons why you couldn't lose five pounds, please don't bother; I have heard all of the excuses. If you lose five pounds in the next two months, I guarantee that you can continue and lose another five pounds in the two following months.

I have a friend who teaches a course in hypnosis for weight control. She says that you should not weigh yourself more than once every two weeks. By doing this, you'll get a better idea of your progress. It is great to see your blood sugar numbers go down while your weight goes down, too. Think of the benefits you'll gain from losing weight. If you are a woman, if you lose 10 pounds, you've just dropped an entire dress size. What if you made a deal with yourself that you would buy one new item of clothing every time you went down a size? Most men couldn't care less, but for us women this is a really big thing. I like new clothing, and it is important to reward ourselves with things that are not food.

Build Strength

You don't have to lift weights all of the time to build strength. Any kind of motion will build strength in different muscles. This is especially important for women after menopause because it strengthens your body and keeps away the risks that come with aging. Osteoporosis, for example, is a serious issue for women, and hip fractures are all too common. Arthritis is also a common occurrence in all aging people.

Does your back ache when you get out of bed in the morning? Don't use that as an excuse. Scientific research and data have shown that following an exercise routine, in moderation and on a regular basis, strengthens the muscles surrounding the joints and protects the joints during movement, making the pains that arise from arthritis lessen. I recommend that you take two bottles of water with you whenever you go walking and hold one in each hand. This adds weight training to walking and helps you lose additional weight. The other thing is that if you drink both bottles by the time you finish your walk, then you have added hydration (fluids) to your body and feel better when you complete your activity.

Improved Insulin Sensitivity

Exercise improves your body's sensitivity to insulin. With improved insulin sensitivity, your insulin works better and because that is happening, you will have lower blood sugar levels, lower insulin levels, and lower A1C levels. All due to exercise! If moving more increases and improves the use of your own insulin and helps deal with the major problem of type 2 diabetes, insulin resistance, then exercise can get you on the way to living better with diabetes.

Improved Blood Sugar Levels

There is no doubt that motion will lower those blood sugar levels. There are all kinds of studies and anecdotal records (stories of people with diabetes) that show that people who increase their activity level often need to have their medications reduced or discontinued. I am making no promises, but it really can make a difference.

Better Psychological Health

When you look better and feel better, you gain a sense of achievement that no one else can give you. Simply feeling better about yourself can in some ways make getting healthier easier. This sense of well-being is very important in order to keep yourself motivated in diabetes self-management.

GETTING STARTED

Before you get started, you need to know where you are. Complete this evaluation of your own day-to-day motion. Doing this will help you take a hard look at your physical activity levels. It may also give you some insight into how

Please answer the following questions.

1. I exercise for 30 minutes a day three times a week ☐ yes ☐ no
2. I play a sport once or twice a week ☐ yes ☐ no
3. I have a job that requires physical activity ☐ yes ☐ no
4. I often walk to my errands instead of driving ☐ yes ☐ no
5. I often play physical games like bowling or golf ☐ yes ☐ no
6. I like to go dancing, swimming, or walking ☐ yes ☐ no
7. I have talked to my doctor about exercise ☐ yes ☐ no
8. I live in an area where I could walk year round ☐ yes ☐ no
9. I think I need to join a gym to exercise ☐ yes ☐ no
10. It is too hard for me to exercise ☐ yes ☐ no

If you answered no to most of the first eight questions and yes to the last two, you are a mudstucker. You are stuck in one position and only a landslide or earthquake makes you move around.

to make some small changes that can really positively affect your blood sugars, weight control, and normal feeling of well-being.

I am not surprised that current data state that 40% of American adults report that they are completely sedentary, which means that a person does not get any significant amount of physical activity in his or her daily life. Dr. Fran Kaufman reports in her book, *Diabesity*, that of the remaining 60% of people who do get some activity, we know that seven out of 10 are somewhat active but fail to meet the recommended standard of activity. Current standards sug-

A Great Role Model

If the discussion about the benefits of physical activity and the problems with getting no activity don't get you into motion, then I have a recommendation for you. Read the story of the governor of Arkansas, Mike Huckabee. He was diagnosed with type 2 diabetes and was vastly overweight. You've probably already heard of him by now. His inspiring story is in the August 2006 issue of *Diabetes Forecast*, and it is the story of a man who took control of his life, his health, and his weight. He lost over 100 pounds and now looks and feels wonderful. Governor Huckabee gives us four great fitness tips that can make motion an important and satisfying part of your daily life.

1. *Make time for physical activity.* Don't find the time; make the time.
2. *Establish a routine.* Set aside a specific routine and build on that.
3. *Pencil it in.* Put exercise on your calendar as you would any other appointment.
4. *Start slowly.* If you do too much too fast, it will turn you off.

Do You Hate to Exercise?

If you, like so many other people, really hate the idea of exercising, there's a great book out there that can help you bring some physical activity into your daily activities around the house and at work. It's called *The "I Hate to Exercise" Book for People with Diabetes*, by Charlotte Hayes.

gest engaging in 30 minutes of strenuous or moderate activity for five or more days a week.

This may seem like a lot of work, but I hope that I have shown that motion doesn't have to be hard to get into and it certainly doesn't have to be boring or a pain. The benefits of exercise are great, and if you have diabetes, you're going to have to get something physical into your daily life.

Ready? Set. Go!

So now that you have decided to move we can talk about getting you started. Please remember that no one should ever start an exercise program without discussing it with his or her doctor. Your doctor may decide that you need a cardiogram before you start running or doing anything, especially if you have been sitting around for years. You see, all people, especially those with diabetes, should have a physical evaluation before beginning an increased level of physical activity. You need to find out what activities are safe.

Your doctor may also recommend an exercise stress test to make sure you are in a good state before you start. You will likely be told to start slowly, and this is good news. Just like losing weight, you can't expect dramatic results right away. Even more, it may not be very healthy. Losing

50 pounds in two months is nearly impossible and dangerous to your health. Likewise, not getting any physical activity and then running a marathon without training can be
equally dangerous. So take things slowly—it's important.

Here is an option that few people are ever told about. Try
asking your health care provider to refer you to a physical
therapist or exercise physiologist, especially if you have physical limitations. These people are trained experts who have
specialized knowledge of how the body works when it is in
physical motion. They can really help you build healthy, safe
activities for your motion plan. People often tell me that they
cannot do anything physical because they have bad knees or
arthritis or are in a wheelchair. There are all kinds of things
that you can do while sitting in a wheelchair to prevent further wasting of muscles or joints, and these professionals can
design this plan. Most insurance companies and Medicare
will pay for this service. It is a shame that so few people are
aware of this wonderful benefit.

YOUR MOTION PLAN

Increasing your activity level is so important for managing
your diabetes that anything you do will make your life
healthier and better. Just do something. Here is a breakdown of things you should know when you start bringing
motion back into your life.

People with diabetes can do all kinds of activities, and
some of the finest athletes in the world have diabetes. A
friend of mine, Olympic gold medalist Gary Hall, is an
inspiration to all people, and the fact that he has diabetes
has never limited him in his dreams and goals. He is a
wonderful man, and I have seen his tireless work in the
cause of diabetes care and education. So, get out there and
have fun! If you love dancing and see me on the dance
floor somewhere, remember to come by and say hello.

General Guidelines

Here are some tips that will keep you safe and healthy while you begin upping your daily physical activity. Remember, though, not to use these as excuses. Don't tell me you can't go walking because you don't have shoes or that it's too hot outside when it's 70 degrees.

Use proper footwear and protective equipment. If you go walking or running without the proper shoes, you can hurt your feet. If you go bicycling without a helmet, what happens if you get into an accident? Make sure you keep yourself safe.

Avoid exercise in extreme heat or cold. Extreme weather conditions can really take their toll on your body, so avoid putting yourself in dangerous situations. You can get dehydrated or suffer heatstroke on hot days, just like you can get frostbitten or ill while out in the cold.

Inspect your feet daily and after exercise. Checking your feet can help you locate wounds in your feet before they turn into ulcers, a terrible complication of diabetes. If you're having trouble with your feet, it's really important to have proper, protective footwear.

Carry identification. You should always wear or carry identification with you when you exercise, and it should always state that you have diabetes. Identification, such as a MedicAlert bracelet, is very important to have for situations when you may need help but can't communicate.

Have water and a carbohydrate snack handy. Dehydration can be a problem when anyone exercises, so keep water handy to solve that problem. Low blood sugar levels (hypoglycemia) can also be an issue while getting physical, so be prepared and have a snack nearby to treat lows.

Physical activity can affect your blood sugar levels in different ways, and it will take some time to become familiar with how activity interacts with your blood sugar levels. Be sure to check your blood sugar before and after exercise, and you may need to stop your activity in the middle, check your blood sugar, have a snack as necessary, and then resume activity. If your blood sugar is high (above 300 mg/dl) before you exercise, don't begin your routine. Wait until your levels are stable, and if your levels stay high, test for ketones in your urine and avoid exercise.

Alternatively, if your blood sugar is low, have a snack before you exercise or you may need to adjust your medication when going on a motion plan. Be sure you get your blood sugar levels to a stable, manageable point before you get going. Talk to your health care provider about how to adjust your medications when you bring motion into your life. More than anything, keep this in mind: if you start to feel funny or strange when you are exercising, slow down and check your blood sugar. It never hurts to be careful.

Different Types of Motion

Aerobic exercise improves your cardiac (heart) and respiratory (lungs) systems, burns calories, and lowers blood sugar levels. Aerobic exercise covers things like jogging, running, swimming, bicycle riding, roller skating, and jumping rope. These are wonderful things to do and some of the most fun.

Strengthening exercises build strong bones and muscles and make your regular routine activities easier. I found that doing laundry and carrying baskets of clothing upstairs was not such a chore after I started lifting weights in the pool. You can do weight training using water bottles, elastic bands, and plastic bags of water or sugar. It's a lot easier to lift the grandchildren after a few months of weight training. If you get a professional to show you how to lift with your legs instead of your back, you will feel a lot better, too.

Flexibility exercises, often called stretching, help keep your joints flexible and are very important in any activity program. Now, you know how I love swimming, so it shouldn't surprise you when I tell you that you can get great benefits from stretching in the pool. It'll provide less wear and tear on your joints, and you'll be surprised at some of the moves you can do in water. You will not believe how great yoga stretching feels in a warm pool.

Warm-up and cool-down periods are essential in any weather and for any activity. You should never neglect warming up and cooling down. In other words, work yourself up and calm yourself down. Warm ups should take 5–10 minutes, and cooling down should take the same

Here's a handy way to think about how to put together your motion plan. The American College of Sports Medicine developed guidelines for an exercise prescription, and I think it's great for people with diabetes. They call it F.I.T.T.

F = Frequency. How often should I exercise without causing stress or damage to my body?

I = Intensity. How hard should I exercise?

T = Type of Exercise. Am I getting all of the different types of activity?

T = Time or Duration. How long should I do the activity?

These are all great questions to think about when it comes to your motion plan. Also, now you see why seeing a doctor, physical therapist, or exercise physiologist is so important. They can help you answer these questions.

amount of time. Both are equally important because they can prevent muscle strains, cramps, and sore bodies. Warm-up and cool-down periods usually include light aerobic exercises, such as jumping jacks, push-ups, and sit-ups (oof!), and flexibility exercises, such as touching your toes, doing arm windmills, and leg stretches.

Walk, Don't Run, to Success

Walking is one of the best things you can do to bring motion into your life, because it can be done anywhere. Remember, walking doesn't burn nearly as many calories as running or rollerblading, so this means that you can't go home and stuff yourself. The best way to start walking is to park your car at the far end of the parking lot and walk. You'll still get your errands done, and you get to top it off with some motion. Anyway, it's better to park far and walk than to spend 20 minutes driving around searching for that one parking place closest to the door.

In many cities there are shopping malls that have walking programs for people who are more comfortable walking indoors or who live in areas where the weather is so nasty that it's nicer being inside. I think mall walking is great fun, and if you do it before the stores open, it can save you a lot of money. One of my favorite forms of motion is walking and shopping. Take the time to find pretty places to walk— places where you get to see new things and new areas. People always tell me that there is nowhere in their neighborhood to walk. It is really all right to drive to a place to take a walk; after all, sometimes walking at a lake, a park, a golf course, or a beach is a lot more interesting and peaceful than walking on a busy sidewalk in a strip mall. Things tend to be more fun if they do not become boring, which means that you are more likely to stick with it. Keeping interest will keep yourself from thinking about your physical activity as a burden.

Exercise Equipment

Many people feel like they should buy exercise equipment to properly do their activities, thinking that this will allow them to maintain a regular schedule. That is really fine if you do actually use that treadmill or rowing machine and don't use it as an expensive clothes rack. There are benefits to having exercise equipment at home, because you can watch television or read while getting yourself into motion. You also get to skip the costs of joining a gym, and weather won't be such a hindrance to your regular schedule. It is also nice to have a set of free weights available if you really enjoy lifting weights. But please remember that you don't need all of this to get your motion plan underway. My attitude toward exercise equipment is that if it's helpful and gets you in shape, then it's perfect, but if it just becomes an obstacle in your spare room or basement, then you've wasted your money and you haven't gotten any closer to becoming fit.

Still, there is a good side to so many people buying exercise gear and never using it. Let me tell you a story from my job. Years ago I wanted to start an exercise program for people with diabetes in a small hospital with limited funds. I put out a notice to the employees and asked people to donate their unused exercise equipment for my program. In a week, I had 10 offers! We wound up with six pieces of equipment that the maintenance department checked and certified as safe for our patients. So, here's a useful lesson to take home: ask your friends and relatives if they have any dusty, unused exercise equipment. You just might find yourself a great treadmill that has been gathering dust for years in someone's basement. You'll also save yourself a lot of money. But before you get started, make sure you have it checked for safety and don't forget to buy your donor a great thank-you gift.

Your Social Life
Eating, Drinking, and Playing

Some of the most important topics to address if you have diabetes are the quality-of-life issues. These are the things that most of us take for granted on a day-to-day basis, such as getting together with friends and family for holidays, birthdays, the birth of children, and the retirement of friends. Some of our favorite memories are those special days that make us smile years later. It may be as simple as sitting around the fire with a glass of wine on a snowy day or the time you scored a hole-in-one on the golf course. Don't let diabetes get in the way of these things. A high quality of life makes life worth living. It would be terrible if you reached a point in your diabetes self-management where you were feeling and doing well but not living well.

Think about the people you know whose lives revolve around going to work, going home, and doing nothing else. I find it hard to consider that living. I used to teach stress classes for health care professionals, and I always asked them what they did every day for themselves. These are people who take care of others day in and day out, and they had a tough time answering that question. They often talked about their favorite things to do on weekends, but the rest of the week was work at work and then work at home. A spouse, kids, housework, and errands can take up every minute of your whole life. If you only "live" for weekends and your days off, then you only live two days a week. I can't afford to waste five days of my life every week. Life is too short.

So let me ask you: what do you do for yourself every day? Do you take an hour to read, watch a favorite show on TV, go for a walk with your friend or spouse, take a bubble bath, play a game, or go to church or other house of worship? These are relaxing moments for you, and no one should live without them, even if he or she has diabetes.

On page 159, there is a chart for you to fill in so you can take a look at your week and examine your priorities. Under each day, enter what you did for yourself last week that was fun or made you feel good. Really think about it. Oh, I have a rule, too. Even if you love your work, you can't put any work activities or job-related duties on this chart. You also can't write in anything you did for someone else. Just write in the things you did for yourself.

After you complete this chart, take a hard look at it. Is there something for you every day? Are there too many blank days with nothing but work and stress and chores but no fun? Do you only work for days off? I hate it when people say, "Thank God it's Friday!" Does that mean that you only live for two days out of the week? Do you just barely survive Monday through Friday? That is sad. Find something—even if it only takes a few minutes each day—that makes you say, "I had a good day today."

Now, take a look at that chart again. Here is something that makes it even more important. You see, having diabetes can be a full-time job. There are no days off, no holidays, and no "just forget about it" days. If you decide to ignore diabetes, it will get even with you. Consider diabetes a selfish lover. You can live with it, but don't live for your blood sugar levels. After all, you're getting healthy so you can enjoy life, not just measure blood sugars.

Sunday	
Saturday	
Friday	
Thursday	
Wednesday	
Tuesday	
Monday	

In this chapter we will examine one of the most important steps of your life, living well, with the full enjoyment of day-to-day living and even year-to-year living. Quality-of-life issues are such an important part of living with diabetes. Talk to your health care provider and diabetes educator and let them help you make the most out of your life. We want to keep you well and living long, but your life also needs to be a good life. You may think of other questions along the way; talk about them. You are entitled to a normal, happy life, and here are some tips for keeping it full and satisfying.

PARTIES, GATHERINGS, AND CELEBRATIONS

Remember that it's good to get out and enjoy your friends and family. Most people use gatherings to do the things that remind them of happy times and to keep up traditions. Parties, gatherings, and celebrations make you think of easier times with fewer responsibilities and of people who may have passed on. Being around these people who are important to your life may remind you of successes or failures in your earlier days, but it always brings back memories. Gathering with loved ones helps us find our place in life, and this is what prepares us for what life holds for us now and in the future.

Eating

Because you now have diabetes, you need to make some plans. Food is a key part of most group events, and all the people who love you will cook and bake what you love to eat and have enjoyed all of your life. Our favorite foods are a comfort in normal life, but because you have diabetes you need to stay in control. People may tell you, or you will tell yourself, that at such celebrations that it's okay for today, just eat right tomorrow. You can't put off eating healthy for tomorrow. It needs to be something you think about every day of your life. Remember, you don't have to eat a different meal than anyone else; you just have to be a little more selective and moderate in your meal planning.

At weddings, for example, people will push food and drinks at you and say things like "It's a wedding; forget the rules for today." That may sound wonderful, but they are not going to feel bad tomorrow. You will. The worst way to celebrate your child's wedding is to make him or her come back from the honeymoon because you are in the hospital. Even though these people mean well, they will not be there when you are sick or in pain from the consequences of taking a day off from your diabetes management. You can have a wonderful time without eating all of the food. Instead, enjoy the activities, the fun, and the special feelings that come from being present at a special day. We often use food to comfort ourselves and make us feel like we are in familiar surroundings. When you are with the people you love, you shouldn't need food to help you feel at home.

One thing that should be a concern when you are at a party or celebration is the time frame. If you are used to eating dinner at 6 p.m. and dinner will not be served until 8 p.m., have a snack at your regular time, but save room for the wonderful dinner planned. Don't forget about the calories that you ate for a snack when you calculate your dinner and make your selections.

You can choose to break away from your normal routines at a party, but remember that you will have to live with the consequences of your decision. Plan ahead. I would rather eat the hors d'oeuvres at a dinner party and not eat all of the full meal. It all comes down to choices. Think about what is going to be served. You may want to skip the pasta and leave room for cake (or at least a taste). At a brunch, you can save a lot of calories by ordering an omelet with vegetables and skipping the hash brown potatoes. Try putting some fruit on the plate and less bread. A handy tip for situations like these is to grab a smaller plate and fill that up; you'll still be eating less than you usually would.

If you are going to a barbecue, make sure there will be some skinless chicken or fish that you can eat and ask about fruit and vegetables. If the only foods are hot dogs, hamburgers, and ice cream, you might want to offer to bring a vegetable platter or plate of chicken or seafood. By doing this, you keep your blood sugars manageable, and you also come across as a gracious guest! Don't forget to watch for all of those unhealthy add-ons at parties. I love going to a great clambake or lobster dinner, but drowning your food in melted butter isn't a good idea. That seven-layer dip might look great and taste even better, but how will you feel the morning after eating a lot of it? You see, it's all about personal choices. It's fine to eat some watermelon, but hold back from eating five wedges. Popcorn can be a healthy alternative to potato chips, but avoid that melted butter. Make sure there will be diet drinks or bring your own. You don't need to make a big stink about it, but it is silly to make yourself sick because you don't want people at the party to know that you have diabetes or because you feel embarrassed bringing something that you can eat.

The holidays take us back to our childhood and the best memories of our youth. A certain cookie may remind you of your grandmother or favorite aunt, and although it really feels good to eat that cookie and relive those memories, the cookie itself is not really good for you. Smell it, taste it, and then put the rest of the cookie in the trash. Save the calories you'd get from eating that whole cookie for healthy foods that will improve your blood sugar levels. Savor these treats, but always remember to do so in moderation.

Many of the American Diabetes Association cookbooks and magazines include holiday recipes that are wonderful, and you might like to share them with your family members. Ask your host or hostess what you can bring to a party. Tell him or her that you have a healthy, great-tasting dish that you would like to share with everyone. You may convert some people into loving healthier foods. As always, though, remember to have fun and enjoy your holidays!

The holiday season can be tough at home, but in some ways, it can be a real trial getting through the holi-

Keeping Your Holidays Healthy

I was director of education in one hospital, and we did a pre-holiday party before Thanksgiving every year. We put out a variety of foods that different people eat around the holiday season and made sure we included food from all cultures. I got to taste wonderful foods from all over the world, and many of my patients proudly shared their favorite dishes with the people they had met in their diabetes support groups.

The dietitian and I escorted each person through the line and helped them make good decisions for a healthy meal plan. We made sure to include their favorite foods and the ones that would be served at their own holiday meals. It was a great success. I suggest that you sit down with the cooks in your family and figure out ways to make those special family dishes healthier and more wholesome. Think about the small changes you can make in the meal that won't really change the ambiance, appearance, or taste but will make it more acceptable to your meal plan.

days at work. Going from department to department at work and eating at each cubicle or office is not a smart health-conscious decision. It's hard to keep track of what you're eating (and therefore track how it will affect your blood sugar levels), and you're almost assured to overeat without knowing it. Candy and treats are everywhere. I used to love working at the hospital at Christmas time. I would make rounds to all of the nursing units and eat all the treats that doctors and the patients' families sent to the staff for the holidays. I was always sick to my stomach by the end of the day, but I still smile when I recall those days.

Physical Activity

If you are going to be dancing at a party, go ahead and eat some more to balance your blood sugar levels, but one slow dance does not equal a full exercise program. If you end up dancing all night, make sure you take a break and test your blood sugars. It really is all right for you to take your meter with you to the party, just put it with your coat and step away for a moment to test.

I know people who never move, but if you find them at a wedding with some music, they'll be on that dance floor all night. The exercise may lower your blood sugar levels, so you may need to stop for a bit and have a snack. The excitement and adrenalin of the party may also raise your blood sugar levels. Testing can be done discreetly and will allow you to feel safe and secure. Doing this will also make your family and friends stop worrying about you and will likely get them off your back. If you are taking a day off from diabetes management, this doesn't mean your loved ones give up caring or worrying about you, so remember to test your blood sugar whether you want to or not. If you can do this, then everyone will be able to enjoy the party.

Remember when you were young and parties were full of physical activities? Maybe it's time to bring that back. Parties always seem to get better when everyone is up and doing something. It can be as simple as tossing that old football around or throwing a pool party. These are great party ideas, especially when you get all of the age groups out there. I hired a square dance caller for my husband's retirement party, and we all danced the night away. I still remember that wonderful time. In fact, I remember it better than a lot of potlucks I've attended.

Drinking Alcohol

If you are going to a party or celebration, odds are that there will be alcohol present. When people with diabetes drink alcohol, there are some basics that you have to know. A glass of wine, a light beer, or a cocktail is fine, but remember to drink in moderation. You have to have good judgment when you have diabetes, and this definitely applies when you combine diabetes and drinking. When

Beverage	Amount	Calories	Carbohydrate (grams)
Light Beer	12 oz	103	6
Regular Beer	12 oz	153	13
Liquor (80 proof)	1 oz	64	0
Liqueur (48 proof)	1 oz	80	9
Wine (white)	5 oz	120	5
Wine (red)	5 oz	129	5

you drink you tend to eat more. The first glass of alcohol will lower your blood sugar levels, so take it with a little food. With that first drink, try to have a cracker or two with a piece of cheese. This will start you off better.

Remember also that when you drink an alcoholic beverage, you're also taking in calories and nutrients. These need to be factored into your meal plan and medication dosages. A 12-ounce glass of light beer has about 103 calories, and a 5-ounce glass of wine has about 129 calories. Remember that alcohol will lower rather than raise your blood sugar, so if you are on insulin you do not need to take extra units when you drink. On page 165 you can see the calories and grams of carbohydrate in some alcoholic beverages. Remember that there are no labels with nutritional data on alcohol, and these numbers are general estimates.

Many companies advertise that their drinks don't contain carbohydrates. They are correct, but don't forget that there are will be calories anyway, just from different sources, such as alcohol. Also remember that if you are drinking, you probably will be munching something as well. Boy, having a drink sure sounds like hard work now, doesn't it?

If you are mixing a cocktail, don't forget the nutritional content of the mixers themselves. If the drink is mixed with a soda, choose a diet soda and check its calories. Most people don't know that you can get a diet tonic instead of a regular one. Try club soda or diet ginger ale as a mixer. An ounce of lime juice has only 8 calories, so a gin and diet tonic with lime juice is a low-calorie cocktail. There is no disgrace with bringing diet tonic to a party or requesting that your host or bartender have some for you.

Scientific data show that a glass or two of wine seems to help prevent heart attacks. You've probably seen and heard this stuff in the news. Most people are pleased when I tell them this or they hear it, but don't forget to count the calories in your meal plan. How about that? I just gave you permission to drink alcohol! For many years, we told patients never to have another beer or drink. They drank anyway but instead tried to hide it from us. I would rather you tell me and your health care providers the truth about your alcohol habits; that way we can help you fit it into your meal plan and give you a plan for making safe, healthy decisions when it comes to drinking. I live in an area where everyone fishes, and the desire to go fishing is only surpassed by the desire to drink a lot of beer. It's pointless for me to tell my patients not to drink, but I can teach them how to reduce

A great rule to follow is to avoid any drink that is served with an umbrella in it. Something has to hold that up, and most of the time it is sugar that does all that heavy lifting. Look for alternatives to thick, sticky drinks. Put an olive in your drink instead of a slice of pineapple. We want you to eat fruit each and every day, but that's a lot of sugar in one sitting. If the drink calls for sugar, use a sugar substitute such as Equal or Splenda. Your drink will taste the same and still give you that kick you love.

their drinking so it does not have any bad effects on their overall health. I spend even more time convincing them to take some food with them and to stick their meter in their tackle boxes.

Remember, moderation is the key to success. You can drink alcohol, just be sure to do it in moderation. Moderation is defined as two drinks a day for men and one drink a day for women. A drink is a 5-ounce glass of wine, a 12-ounce light beer, or 1 1/2 ounces of 80-proof distilled spirits (liquor). Make sure that your medications don't require avoiding alcohol, and get your doctor's okay.

TRAVELING WITH DIABETES

When planning a vacation, think about how you are going to travel with your supplies. Never leave your medications, syringes, or meters in a checked suitcase. These must be carried by hand and be available at all times. Remember that luggage gets lost all the time, and even a short delay can be serious if your medication is in the bag. Always carry prescriptions for your medications, strips, syringes, needles, lancets, or anything else you use. Sometimes airlines require that you show them these prescriptions before they will allow you on a plane with a syringe and needle. It is a good idea to check with your airline and find out what they require from you. You should also check to see what the latest requirements are for federal aviation security by visiting the website for the U.S. Transportation Security Administration at www.tsa.gov. Having your needles confiscated by a security guard would be a horrible way to start a vacation. We want to be safe when traveling, so take the extra time to be prepared.

This is especially true when you are traveling out of the country. If you are applying for a visa, or your travel agency is doing it for you, make sure you put on the visa that you have diabetes and will be traveling with all kinds of supplies. I suggest you carry double the amount of supplies and medication that you think you will need for the trip. You can always carry it home, so what is the big deal if you have to lug around a few extra supplies? If you are going to a country where English is not the primary language, find out how to say "I have diabetes" in that language and write it down.

Here's an example from my life. I was in Glasgow, Scotland, on September 11, 2001. After those terrible events, we could not get home for five more days, which caused much concern for the group that was there for the conference of the European Association for the Study of Diabetes. There were thousands of us from the U.S., and many of the group had diabetes. I had taken only enough blood pressure medication to last the trip and two extra days, so it became a real issue when I started running low on my pills. The conference arranged to have a local doctor write prescriptions for us and fill them, so this large group of health care professionals would not find themselves in trouble. You may not be so fortunate if you find yourself in the same situation.

Don't forget about changing time zones, either. It is always a good idea to sit down with your doctor or diabetes educator and discuss how to revise the times when you should take your medications when you cross time zones.

Think about what you would do if you found yourself somewhere during a hurricane, like Wilma, and were stranded for over 10 days without extra supplies and medications. It could become an emergency situation and even be life threatening. Please remember that if there is a power outage, then you also lose refrigeration. There are cool packs that activate only when you smash them on a hard surface, so these can be packed in your suitcase to keep your insulin cool. I highly recommend that you carry them when you travel. It is always better to be safe than sorry.

Whenever you travel anywhere, bring identification that shows that you have diabetes. People have been arrested because police who were unfamiliar with the signs of diabetes mistakenly thought these people were intoxicated instead of suffering from a low blood sugar. You need to have some kind of alert bracelet or identification on you at all times. A wallet card that shows you have diabetes and the name of a family member or doctor is the absolute minimum that you should carry.

Some countries and U.S. states restrict what fruits, vegetables, and other produce you can take with you on an airplane. For example, both Florida and California will not allow you to transport foreign fruit into their borders. You may be allowed to take them on the plane, however, as long as you eat them onboard or dispose of them before leaving the place. Dried fruits and nuts are really great travel foods and are good substitutes for fresh fruit.

You should always carry food in case you are delayed and have quick sugar sources for long flights or car trips. Many airlines allow you to preorder a "diabetic diet," but these won't be necessary if you are prepared by carrying your own food so you can adapt the food to your meal plan. If you expect the airline to have the right food for your meal plan, you may be very disappointed and find yourself hungry halfway through the flight. I recently took a train trip that was supposed to take nine hours, and instead, it wound up taking 16 hours. I have been on airplanes that circled for three hours or sat on the runway for hours, and no one could serve us food because we were in an active pattern. Does this sound familiar? If it does, then this should show you how important it is to be prepared.

You can travel safely and successfully if you plan ahead and take some simple precautions. If you are not comfortable with this process, start by talking to your diabetes educator or physician. If you are planning a major trip, I suggest that you think of a travel agent instead of doing it yourself. You have more things to consider than ordinary travelers, including health care, food choices, and traveling with medications, and a good travel professional may provide great support for your travel plans. If you do decide to follow this advice, make sure the agent you choose is familiar with international travel and has experience planning trips for people with diabetes.

A Handy Travel Reference

If you're looking for some great in-depth information on how to travel with diabetes, you should take a look at this wonderful book, *The Diabetes Travel Guide*, by Davida Kruger. It has a ton of information, including a nice little phrasebook in the back that can tell you how to tell people that you have diabetes in many different languages.

Long trips don't just happen on airplanes and trains. You can take really long trips in the car, too, and you need to be prepared on those trips as well. Please think about putting a diabetes box or kit in your car. I like to put emergency supplies in my trunk because you never know what can happen. This kit should include a spare meter, strips, glucose tablets, peanut butter crackers, and medications. Be sure to check that these supplies are not sensitive to extreme temperatures that may arise in cars. Also, don't forget that wherever you go, you are the person who should carry a cell phone. In the event of an emergency it is important that you can get help. Program your family, doctor, emergency services, and the person you trust most into the phone, so you can reach them quickly.

If this sounds like a lot of bother, it isn't. These little tasks are absolutely worth your time and energy. I hope you never need the supplies in your emergency kit. It probably won't be used in your day-to-day life, but it will be there for those long car trips and for the short ones when something might go wrong.

SEXUALITY

Now let's discuss your sexual life. Many people with diabetes enjoy a healthy sexual life, and there is no reason that should not apply to you. Everyone needs to know that someone loves and cares about them and that their loved one will be there for them during every stage of their life. Sometimes that assurance is more important than the sexual activity itself. You may, upon being diagnosed with diabetes, find yourself distracted, worried, or upset, which certainly might take your mind off sex for a while. Don't forget that your partner may be just as upset as you are to find out that you have diabetes and an upset partner can also affect your sex life. Do not be embarrassed about discussing sex, because these issues are every bit as important as any of the other problems that go hand and hand with diabetes.

It always amazes me when health care providers are hesitant to discuss sexual issues with patients unless the patient brings it up. A person's sexual life is incredibly important, so you, as a person with diabetes, should always feel free to bring up this topic with your health care providers. It can be easy to become frightened or depressed, but your health

An important issue is personal attractiveness. A person can grow to fear that his or her body, perhaps because of weight issues, makes him or her unattractive to a loved one. It is hard to think about sex when you are feeling dumpy, frumpy, old, and miserable because you just found out you have diabetes and someone told you that you have to lose 50 or 100 pounds. It is also hard to be attracted to a person who is nagging you about eating all the time and making you feel like you have no willpower or self-control. Does this sound familiar? If so, start dealing with the issue by talking to your diabetes educator. Sometimes just starting the conversation gets you on track for solving the problem. No one should let diabetes make them feel like they are undesirable.

care providers are there to make sure that you are able to effectively cope with this. It's simple to get a referral to a gynecologist or urologist, but you should never be afraid to bring up your concerns. Remember what I've been telling you, you are the captain of your ship. If your health care team does not address your sexual life, you have a right to insist that this important topic be discussed.

For Women

Diabetes sometimes presents physical sexual issues for women, so there are some things to think about. Years ago, women with type 1 diabetes were told to avoid getting pregnant and that pregnancy could possibly be life threatening. This is no longer the case, but young people with diabetes should be taught about the importance of good blood sugar management and planning for pregnancies. Nowadays, people with diabetes do very well and have normal, healthy, beautiful babies just like everyone else. Some people who have difficult pregnancies are encouraged to see physicians who handle high-risk pregnancies. If you have type 1 diabetes and are contemplating pregnancy, you

Teenagers and Sex

Teenagers with diabetes should have sexual counseling so they can avoid the risks of an unplanned pregnancy. Adolescence is not the time to avoid conversations about safe sex and birth control. People of all cultures and religions have methods of dealing with pregnancies, and diabetes should not get in the way of this. In fact, if a teen has diabetes, then this issue absolutely must be discussed with honesty and frankness.

should always work with a team that includes an endocrinologist and a gynecologist, both of whom should have experience with diabetes.

Female sexual issues are not as visible as those of men, so they are not often discussed. In addition, women are often afraid to discuss sex with male doctors. You may be more

Talking Can Help

I once had a patient who was being discharged from the hospital after having a hysterectomy, which is a surgery in which the uterus and sometimes the cervix are removed. She was very worried about how she would feel as a sexual woman after this surgery and about how her husband would think of her. On the day of discharge, I accompanied a student nurse into the room to see if this patient had been adequately prepared for discharge. The patient's husband was at her side, and he was very interested in the discussion. Near the end of the conversation, I asked the patient if the student nurse had discussed when they could resume sexual activities and to what extent. The patient blushed, and the student turned white and hemmed and hawed. The topic had not come up, so I went into the whole process.

At the end of the conversation I asked if either of them had any questions before they were ready to go. The husband took his wife's hand, kissed it, and said that if he knew things were going to be so good, he would have made the doctor discharge her earlier. She smiled and kissed him back. When they left they were a close couple that felt good about themselves and their ability to get through this life-changing procedure. The lesson for you is to make sure that you get the knowledge, information, and instruction that you need to be comfortable with life. A little bit of embarrassment isn't worth feeling terrible if you don't have to.

comfortable discussing it with a gynecologist or diabetes educator. Young women can have irregular periods or not menstruate at all, so it is important to get the accurate facts from a health care professional and not the rumor mill. Things always seem worse when you hear about them from a neighbor who read about the problem in a magazine article.

We know that there are physical problems, such as vaginal dryness or painful intercourse. We also know that there may be menstrual changes, worries about pregnancy, and chemical changes in your body that cause yeast infections. Somehow these things do not get discussed in diabetes classes or with your doctor unless you bring them up or are having one of these problems. Too often, I find out that my patients are depressed and feel like they're the only ones in the world with these problems. They aren't, and neither are you. So please speak up.

For Men

Some men do find that they have some problems with sexual performance. Erectile dysfunction (also called impotence) is sometimes an issue with people with poorly controlled blood sugar levels. If you can properly manage your blood sugar levels, then you can usually avoid this problem. If you do find that you have erectile dysfunction, there are many successful treatments. Make sure you talk to your doctor, and don't be ashamed to admit that you need some assistance. Having erectile dysfunction because of diabetes is not a disgrace. In fact, it is much more common than people want to admit. You may ask your doctor to refer you to a urologist who can discuss the different ways to deal with the issue. The worst thing you can do is to ignore the situation and hope it will go away. It won't; in fact, it will likely worsen.

New medications, such as Viagra (generic name, sildenafil citrate), Levitra (generic name, vardenafil), and Cialis (generic name, tadalafil), increase the blood flow to the penis, thus allowing an erection. These medications have been found to be very successful in a large number of patients. However, like with all medications, there are side effects and safe use of these drugs should be discussed with your physician.

There are other methods of dealing with erectile dysfunction. They include injections or suppositories that are applied directly to the penis and even an implanted penile prosthesis. This last treatment requires that a vacuum device be inserted into the penis, and a pump inflates the device, giving the person an erection.

CONCLUSION

We have only discussed some of the quality-of-life issues. However, lots of people value different things when they assess their quality of life. What if skydiving or flying airplanes is really important to you, for instance? Well, you should talk to someone about the restrictions that may change this. You may have to find something to do that diabetes does not hinder or restrict by law.

You will notice that I did not even discuss smoking because there is no way I can agree with you or suggest a compromise if you decide to keep smoking. It is so dangerous for people with diabetes to smoke. There are many alternatives available to help you give up this dangerous habit. Talk to your diabetes educator or look for smoking cessation courses in your area. There are always options on the Internet as well. Please consider this. Quitting smoking can instantly improve your quality of life.

Seven

The Financial
Side of Diabetes

Let's talk about another important issue that will help you deal with the diabetes life you now live. It is not as emotional as finding out that you have diabetes but may be as worrisome as any other part of your care and planning. We're going to talk about the finances involved in managing your diabetes.

Let's take a look at the number of things you have to think about when you have diabetes: meal planning, medications, monitoring, and keeping yourself motivated. Now throw in worrying about paying for everything. This is a lot to think about, but it's not a problem that can't be overcome. The financial side of diabetes is a major issue for everyone, and the entire diabetes community spends a lot of time trying to help people with diabetes deal with money problems. I know that this can be very frustrating, and I am sure you worry about how much this thing is going to cost now and for the rest of your life. Still, keep in mind that stress will raise your blood sugar levels, so make reasonable plans on how to deal with your finances. If you can do this, you won't have to spend all of your energy worrying about money.

I advise you to look at the alternatives covered in this chapter and to select the one that is relevant to your life.

Then think about the advice I've given you and talk to someone who is capable and available to help you with your financial plans. Make sure that you include your significant other in these discussions, so he or she can know what is happening and can handle the issue if you are ill or too busy to deal with the finances. You don't have to read the sections that are not important to you now, but please take a glance at them and remember where they are just in case there is a change in your health care status. For example, you may be employed now and covered by your employer's group insurance, but when you hit 65 years of age, you will be eligible for Medicare. This constitutes a major change in costs and coverage. You should also know that the rules governing Medicare and Medicaid change almost every year, so it is important that you keep aware of what is happening in the financial world of diabetes care. You can always find the most current information at the advocacy or reimbursement section of the American Diabetes Association website (www.diabetes.org). If you are not a computer person, you can call them at 1-800-DIABETES.

The Costs of Diabetes

A study from 2003 showed us that the cost of health care for people with diabetes is about $13,243 per person per year. For people who don't have diabetes, their costs are $2,560 per person per year. These figures include days missed at work, plus those due to disability. A chronic disease costs money. Because you cannot decide to stop taking your medications this month (that would be very dangerous), you need to find ways to pay for your diabetes costs. The American Diabetes Association estimates that over $132 billion was spent on diabetes-related care in 2006, and the projected costs of the future are constantly increasing.

There are several different ways to pay for diabetes care, and I want to tell you about them and give you some resources to help. Some of this can be very complicated, but we will go over all of the options so you can see which one works best for you.

KEEPING RECORDS CAN SAVE CASH AND KEEP YOU ORGANIZED

The first thing to think about is how much you will be relying on the health care system. You will be making regular doctor visits more often than most people. People with type 1 diabetes often see both their primary care physicians and their endocrinologists several times a year. People with type 2 diabetes often see their doctors at least twice a year and often four times a year. You may decide to visit a podiatrist for regular foot exams and wound prevention. You will now have to be more conscious about getting flu shots every year and having blood tests as recommended. Does it sound like I am spending your time as well as your money? Well, I am, because diabetes requires full-time attention. It will be a good idea to keep a calendar to record and keep track of your medical office visits, lab work, and routine check-ups.

Here's an example from my life. My husband was diagnosed with cancer in 2003. He's fine now, thank goodness, but I learned the importance of keeping good records from the experience. I kept a running log of doctor visits, treatments, tests, and lab work and results on the computer, which I updated after each visit. Entries were logged in chronological (by date) order and very easy to follow. Each time we went to the doctor, I brought them a copy of the log for their reference, and it saved us a lot of time, energy, and money because none of the treatments or tests was needlessly repeated. Make sure you get copies of all of your lab work, X-rays, and other diagnostic tests and take them with you on visits, so you can also avoid having different health care providers repeating the same tests on you. It will save you a lot of anger, frustration, and co-pays. Keep track of absolutely everything you have to do, have already done, and will have to do that involves health care providers, costs, and diabetes.

I am enclosing a sample of a medical record that you can use for yourself. Just copy and fill in the blanks. Always bring this with you when to go to medical visits.

Private Health Care Record

Name_____ Date Started_____

Date	Doctor	Lab work	Diagnostic tests	Comments
6/06/06	Smith-Clark	Blood test, urine test, A1C	Chest X-ray	Medications changed. To see Doctor in September. To see Podiatrist. A1C is 7.8%. All other tests negative.

I keep this chart on my computer and fill it in after every visit to a doctor. At the next visit, I print it out, bring it to the office, and hand it to whichever health care professional we are visiting. It makes a lot a sense and saves you so many headaches. It is also helpful to keep a chart like this if you have to send your records to

Medicare or your insurance company. I like to staple copies of the lab work to the back. This way, I know we always have the records, even if the doctor's office misplaces their files. Be sure to keep a folder for all of this stuff and make sure your family knows where to find it.

Get Free Information at Conventions and Health Fairs

You will hear about exhibits and health fairs, and I suggest you go and look at what is out there in the world of diabetes. The more you know about the diabetes world you live in, the more you will be interested in taking care of yourself and keeping your care as current as possible. I am often invited to speak at these conventions, so I regularly find myself astounded at the new drugs and equipment that are being developed to make your life easier and better. At our annual meeting an entire convention center level is full of exhibits from all of the pharmaceutical companies and medical equipment manufacturers. You get to talk to the very knowledgeable people who work the booths and can answer all kinds of questions. You actually get an opportunity to look, handle, and try the equipment yourself. You also will have an opportunity to collect samples and helpful educational materials. I always go with an empty suitcase to bring back samples and materials that I can give to my patients and colleagues. Even though many of these events are for diabetes professionals, you might want to go to one anyway, just to see what it's like.

More importantly, you will have an opportunity to listen to wonderful speakers who have information that will be helpful when you have to make choices about your care. There is something else that may be very helpful: it's called networking. Talk to other people in the meetings and classes. They will be very willing to discuss their lives and experiences with you and become a part of your diabetes support system.

PRIVATE HEALTH INSURANCE

If you are like most people, the world of health insurance can be very confusing. It is not always clear what is covered or what can be reimbursed. Policies can be very confusing, and when you are dealing with a chronic disease, it is important that you keep your knowledge up to date on your insurance status. You need to learn the language of insurance to understand what it really means. Don't be embarrassed if you don't understand the terminology because there's no way to learn except by asking what these strange words mean. I often teach classes for doctors and managed-care plan employees, and I beg them to put their insurance terms in simple English. I sometimes feel like this may be a losing battle, but perhaps if we all work together, some changes will be made and health insurance doesn't have to sound like it comes from a foreign language.

There are many kinds of health care policies, and they all pay for certain things and not for others. If you are employed, your company may pay for your health insurance in total or in part and then you have to pay the rest. It may cover you or your entire family, depending on how much you pay. Most company policies are for large groups of employees, which means that you may have more benefits because lots of people are in the group and this spreads the costs. Then there are private health insurance policies, in which you pay for all of the insurance for yourself and your family. Take it from me, a private policy is always more expensive than a group plan.

Sometimes, companies provide health insurance to employees who retire. If that is ever offered to you, seriously consider it because it is a wonderful benefit. If your children are covered by your policy, they are usually covered until they reach their 18th birthday or when they graduate from school, whether that means from high school, from college, or joining the armed forces. Make sure you know what your company considers the last date of eligibility for your children.

The Basics

If your insurance is through your employer you can discuss the policy with your benefits coordinator at your job, and he or she will explain and clarify your benefits. Some jobs will offer you a choice of different kinds of policies, and you must really understand what you are choosing and how much it will cost you. Often the benefits coordinator will offer educational sessions explaining all of the choices and will sit down with you to help you choose. Do not be embarrassed to ask for help. This is what these people get paid to do, and I think they are the only ones who really know what is going on. Sometimes representatives of the insurance company will come to these sessions and stay to answer questions. Remember that they are used to using the jargon of their business, but don't be afraid to ask them to translate what they are saying into plain English.

Your benefits person can also be especially helpful when your insurance company does not respond to your needs. You may feel that your insurance company is not paying for what you need and for what you believe should be covered. Remember that your benefits coordinator pays the bills for the insurance and negotiates contracts, so he or she has more clout when dealing with the insurance company.

Employers want you stay healthy, because they have finally discovered that it pays to cover preventive care, doctor's visits, screenings, and vaccinations rather than to have you miss days from work or spend time in hospitals. Many companies sponsor health fairs and wellness programs. These are often educational sessions set up on a regular basis for employees and their family members. This trend

You will be taking various medications, testing your blood, and using many other supplies made for people with diabetes. Often your health care providers will tell you what you should be using, but you will also be surrounded by hundreds of advertisements for all sorts of interesting and exciting things available to people with diabetes. There are some great things out there, but you should always remember that there will be things you need, things you will want, and things that are just nice, interesting, or fun to have. Please remember, before you buy all those fancy bells and whistles, make sure you know how you will be paying for the things that you absolutely have to pay for, like your pills and/or insulin.

toward preventive care has become more common over the past decade, and there are all kinds of data available to prove that these programs keep people healthy and save businesses millions of dollars in medical care and insurance payments over the long term.

When an insurance company issues you a policy they will give you a membership card. Put it in your wallet and always carry it. You can request an extra card from the company to leave at home in your medical file. There will be a toll-free number on the back that is absolutely essential for your coverage and care. Sometimes you will receive a separate card just for medications. If you have several cards, carry them all. I recommend that you make copies of your cards; give a set to your spouse and leave a copy at home. Losing your wallet is hard enough, but keeping these copies gives you some security while you get your cards replaced. This can often take several weeks, and if you don't have copies of your cards, you may not have the phone numbers and membership numbers you need to request replacement cards.

Build a Relationship with Your Insurance Company

I suggest that you call the insurance company and establish a relationship with your managed-care coordinator so you can feel comfortable and confident with your insurance company before you have any problems. Make an introductory call on a calm, quiet day. I have found that you should avoid calling on Mondays and Fridays because those are always the busiest and most stressful days at work. Avoid lunchtime, too, as the phone lines are busy, and people get impatient and testy when they are busy and stressed. Be prepared to wait and have everything you need in front of you. You will need your membership cards, a list of your medications and equipment, and your doctor's numbers and address. Ask for your managed-care representative or coordinator, and when you get that person ask for his or her name and number, so you can call them directly next time.

Tell them who you are and explain that you are calling to introduce yourself and explain your care requirements. Tell them that you are prepared to take care of yourself by visiting your doctor, taking your medications, testing your blood sugars, and doing all the things necessary to stay well and avoid complications. Tell them that you will be saving them a lot of money for hospitals and care by taking care of yourself and that you expect them to be your partner in this plan by paying for what you need and by allowing you to be a partner with your health care team. I have found that this conversation really pays off and allows you to reduce the stress involved in dealing with health insurance. Your insurance providers and employers really want you to stay well and are often pleased to work with you to clear up any misunderstandings about your benefits.

If you wait until you have a problem and call when you are upset or angry, the chances that anything will be solved are slim to none. You will be just another angry, nasty, or dissatisfied customer who is ruining their day. An important thing to understand is that it can be very difficult for these insurance representatives to deal with angry, frustrated customers, so try to be patient and understanding when you're calling because of a problem. If you think you are covered for something but are not sure, call the toll-free number and get "pre-certified." This means that you get permission from the insurance company to get the service before you go for the visit or procedure. This can save you a lot of aggravation and is well worth the time you spend calling.

When you look at a policy, look at the choices. Some companies offer a menu of benefits and let you select what you need and allow you to give up unnecessary benefits. A great example is giving up maternity benefits when you hit fifty and instead adding disability or life insurance.

Eligibility for Insurance

Many people with diabetes are concerned that they might not be eligible for insurance because they have diabetes and it is considered a "preexisting condition." Although it is true that some companies may turn you down, many others will cover you.

The American Diabetes Association has an advocacy committee that has been working for years to establish health care insurance rights for people with diabetes. In 2005, a bill was introduced in the U.S. Senate that would allow insurance companies to opt out of covering diabetes education and supplies in many states. A concentrated effort was launched to lobby senators to defeat the bill. We were successful! For now, the right to health insurance for people with diabetes is safe. However, you should stay informed about new developments in health care issues in your federal, state, and local governments. Proposed legal changes may directly affect what will or will not be paid for in diabetes care. I highly recommend that you contact the American Diabetes Association at 1-800-DIABETES or go online to www.diabetes.org and look at the advocacy section for developments in your area. Or you can simply type the word "insurance" into the search box.

COBRA

If you change jobs, you are eligible for COBRA, which is short for the Consolidated Omnibus Budget Reconciliation Act. The rules behind COBRA say you must be covered under your employer's policy for 18 months after you leave your job. If you are disabled, it may be for a longer period of time. You have to pay the insurance premiums, but they are usually cheaper than if you have to get coverage on your own. COBRA gives you time to arrange insurance through your new job. Many employers say that you have to work for them for three to six months before they will cover you with their employee plans, so COBRA allows you to deal with that gap. It is an excellent benefit.

One last piece of advice: check with your benefits coordinator if you ever have questions. Don't ask your co-workers for technical answers to your insurance coverage questions. They can be right, but when they are wrong, I've found that people can give terrible misinformation that causes all kinds of difficulties. This is a pretty good rule for everything. People are so anxious to show you how smart they are that they often make it seem like they are experts when they really don't know much of anything. Please, go to the experts when you have questions because your health requires correct information.

NO HEALTH INSURANCE?

If you are one of the 40 million Americans who have no health insurance at all and are not eligible for Medicaid or Medicare, you have big problems. It is often difficult to make choices about what you can pay for, and sometimes diabetes supplies may not make it to the top of your list. If this situation applies to you, have a frank discussion with your health care provider and explain your difficulties.

I have worked with durable medical equipment companies in the past, and they always set aside equipment for patients who cannot pay for diabetes meters or supplies. A durable medical equipment company sells or rents medical supplies, such as meters and strips, and larger medical equipment, such as hospital beds, wheelchairs, respiratory equipment, and home care items, to the public. They are experts in the field of reimbursement and can help you get what you need at the best prices or help you complete the forms that will get your equipment paid for by Medicare or your insurance company. They usually have case workers who will do all of the paperwork for you. These companies and pharmaceutical companies often get bad press, but they are also very generous to people who need help to survive diabetes. Contact the company that makes your medication and ask for the patient assistance service or patient assistance line. Companies often try to help patients by giving them medications at reduced prices or at no charge, but you have to call this service to get it. Try calling 411 or directory assistance and ask for the toll-free numbers for the drug companies that make your medications and supplies. In chapter 10, I have given you the numbers for some pharmaceutical and equipment companies to save you time.

Many physicians will help patients with medication samples and testing strips. Diabetes educators often give patients supplies and materials sent to them from pharmaceutical companies. No one wants patients to suffer or to have to choose between eating every day and taking their medications. All of us in the diabetes community will do whatever we can to assist you in your care.

Getting Support

It is important that you look into the social services that may be available to you from the community in which you live. Look in the telephone book, usually in the front of the guide, for government services. You should be able to find the numbers for professionals who know the services available for you in your area and who can refer you to social services. Try calling the services for the aging office in your area for assistance. Also, don't forget that every hospital has a social service department to help patients. If you are hospitalized, please make sure to talk to the discharge planning department and see how they can help you get in touch with the agencies you need.

Recently, I watched a case worker interview a patient who had just been discharged from major surgery. She asked him about the stairs in his home, about disability payments from his job, and if he wanted a home care worker to help him with his housework while he was recuperating. I was very impressed and very pleased. You may not get this kind of case worker, even though it is available, so never hesitate to seek out help. The worst thing you can do is to not get something you need and suddenly find yourself in real physical trouble. Get someone to help you. You do not have to do this alone.

There are community and religious groups that help people obtain services that they cannot afford. Groups like

The Partnership for Prescription Assistance

There is a service, started in 2005, called the Partnership for Prescription Assistance Program. It is made up of American pharmaceutical companies, doctors, other health care providers, patient advocacy groups, and community groups. It helps qualifying patients who lack prescription coverage receive the medications they need through public or private programs. You can find out more about this program by going to their website at www.pparx.org or call 1-888-4PPA-NOW (1-888-477-2669). At this site you will be asked what medications you are taking, and it will give you a list of options to obtain them at lower prices or sometimes free of charge.

the Lion's Club, Rotary Club, Community Chest, and United Way spend their time trying to assist people in obtaining the care and help they very much need. If you are homebound, you may be eligible for a meal-delivery service or food stamps that will help pay for some of your expenses. You might want to ask a member of your local clergy what services exist in your community. These people are very knowledgeable and stay informed about services that are available to their parishioners. Sometimes there will be a group that provides rides to the doctor's office, and joining a group like that can save you enough transportation money to spend on your medications. Last, talk to the people in your town hall and find out if you are eligible for a reduced tax rate because of your age or because you have a chronic disease like diabetes.

MEDICARE

If you are age 65 or older or have been on disability leave, then you are entitled to Medicare coverage. This is a federal

program, and you may hear it called Medicare Part A or
Part B. In 1997 the Budget Reconciliation Act added diabetes education and supplies to the list of treatments eligible for Medicare reimbursement. The entire diabetes community was thrilled that we would see major changes in
benefits for people with diabetes.

Unfortunately, this act did not, as most people believed,
make all diabetes supplies and medications covered by
Medicare. Only meters, strips, lancets, and a major program
of diabetes education are covered. We are still grateful for
this amount of coverage because it is a major benefit that
continues to change. I was at the event with President
Clinton when he announced the coverage change. It was
truly an exciting day of all of us who care for people with
diabetes or have diabetes.

If you are not taking insulin you are allowed 100 glucose-
testing strips every three months, but if you take insulin
you can get 100 per month. In either case, your doctor can
write a letter or fill out a waiver form if he or she feels you
need more strips to test more often. As long as your health
care provider can justify the need in writing, Medicare will
probably pay for more supplies.

Over the last few years Medicare has added new services, such as insulin pumps and therapeutic shoes, if you
qualify. Remember to get prescriptions for everything you
need. In January 2006, prescription drugs were added to
Medicare services (called Plan D), which include insulin,
syringes, and diabetes medication.

If you have Medicare you are eligible for 10 hours of
diabetes self-management education from a certified diabetes education program that is approved by the American
Diabetes Association. You must get a referral from your
physician or primary care provider in order to get Medicare
to pay for the program, so don't be afraid to ask about it.
I have constantly encouraged you to attend a diabetes

self-management education course, so I won't badger you any further here.

You can also see a registered dietitian for three hours of medical nutrition therapy. Taking advantage of this benefit will help you learn how to manage a meal plan. This is a very important service and is separate from the full 10-hour diabetes self-management education course. After your first year of Medicare coverage, you will be covered for an additional two hours with the dietitian.

If you have nerve damage in your feet, you should have a foot exam by a podiatrist every six months, and Medicare also covers this. You do not need a prescription from your doctor for this service. You are also covered for a dilated eye exam to check for retinopathy or other diabetes eye problems.

As of January 2005, a wonderful benefit was added for you and your family members who become eligible for Medicare for the first time. There is now a "Welcome to Medicare" physical. This is a one-time physical assessment to review of all your health needs. It will assess your need for preventive care, screenings, vaccinations, and treatments. It also includes diabetes screening, blood tests, and glaucoma screening, which can prevent blindness before it starts. This wonderful benefit must be used within the first six months that you are eligible for Medicare. Remember to schedule these appointments quickly because if you don't use them, you lose them. To be eligible for the diabetes screening, you must meet some specific criteria, such as high blood pressure, high cholesterol, obesity, heart disease, or family members with diabetes. You are also covered for flu and pneumonia injections. As a person with diabetes this is absolutely required for a healthy lifestyle.

Remember, every year, in January, you will have to pay a deductible of about $100 for your health care, and then Medicare will pay for 80% of your covered care, education,

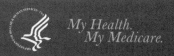

★ ★ TIP SHEET ★ ★

Information Partners Can Use on:

Important Updates to Medicare's Diabetes-related Covered Services in 2007

As of November 2006

Medicare is committed to identifying and treating people with diabetes more effectively. In 2005, we expanded coverage for preventive services to include diabetes screening. Starting January 1, 2007, Medicare will provide more coverage for services that affect people with diabetes. Below are the highlights of the changes that may affect people with Medicare with or at risk for diabetes.

- Medicare will increase payment to doctors for the most frequently billed face-to-face doctor/patient service. This service includes instances where the doctor and patient discuss the patient's health and what needs to be done to maintain or improve their health. We believe this will help to encourage more discussions about controlling diabetes. This includes referring more of the eligible patients to other qualified providers for Medicare-covered preventive services like diabetes outpatient self-management training and medical nutrition therapy.

- Medicare is expanding access to rural and underserved areas. Diabetes outpatient self-management training and medical nutrition therapy services will be covered services included in the Federally Qualified Health Center benefit. For more information on Federally Qualified Health Centers, visit http://www.cms.hhs.gov/center/fqhc.asp on the web.

- Medicare is updating a broad range of preventive services, including adding a new abdominal aortic aneurysm screening to the "Welcome to Medicare" physical exam and excluding colorectal cancer screening procedures from the Part B deductible.

Medicare pays for many preventive services to help keep people healthy. Encourage people with Medicare to get the most out of their Medicare benefits and take advantage of the preventive services available to them to help improve their quality of life. While preventive services generally include exams, lab tests, and screenings, they also include shots, monitoring, and information to help people take care of their own health.

For a complete list and details of Medicare's preventive services, visit www.medicare.gov on the web and select "Preventive Services," or get a free copy of "Guide to Medicare's Preventive Services" by selecting "Publications." You can also call 1-800-MEDICARE (1-800-633-4227) for more information. TTY users should call 1-877-486-2048.

Encourage people with Medicare to register at MyMedicare.gov to gain access to personalized information regarding Medicare benefits and services, including eligibility, entitlement and preventive services they may be eligible for.

CMS Pub. No. 11274-P is printed with the permission of the Centers for Medicare & Medicaid Services.

and supplies. This means that you are responsible for the other 20% of your costs, which have to be paid out of pocket. *Please know that this deductible changes every year.* You should check with your doctors, pharmacists, or supplier to see if they will accept Medicare assignment, which means they will only charge you what Medicare pays and not the additional 20%.

In a newsletter from Medicare, you are encouraged to get a copy of a booklet, *Medicare Coverage of Diabetes Supplies & Services.* You can call Medicare at 1-800-MEDICARE or visit their website at www.medicare.gov. This particular booklet is publication #11022.

I highly recommend, if you can afford it, that you consider supplementary health insurance. These policies from AARP, Oxford, Blue Cross/Blue Shield, and others will pay for your out-of-pocket expenses, deductibles, and other things that are not covered. Please take the time to consider the advantages of supplementary health insurance because it can save you a lot of money.

Medigap

There is also a program called Medigap that you should know about. This is a supplemental insurance policy for Medicare beneficiaries designed to fill in the gaps of Medicare Plans A and B. It is sold by private insurance companies, so you will have to pay a monthly premium if you choose to go with this option. There are many different Medigap policies, and each has a different set of benefits. It is very helpful to have Medigap coverage, but you have to be very careful when you select a plan. Monthly premiums can differ from one provider to the next. These policies may help pay health care costs, but only if you already have the original Medicare. You cannot be turned down if you apply during the first six months that you have Medicare, but if you wait you may have to meet certain medical requirements to be accepted.

MEDICAID

Medicaid is a benefit that began in 1966 under title 19 of the Social Security Act. It is intended to help people who have a low income and no health insurance. Although it is a federal program, local state governments administer and run their own Medicaid programs. Each state determines what it will pay for in a specific area. People must apply for Medicaid, and requirements differ in each area.

In your home state there is a program attached to Medicare called SHIP or State Health Insurance Assistance Program. Look for it in the phone book. These programs have trained counselors who will talk to you directly about your Medicare options and are familiar with the rules and regulations of your specific area.

Medicaid will pay for medical treatment at all levels and has been very helpful in providing payment for attendance in diabetes self-management education programs. If you have questions about this service in your area, look at the state or county government pages of your phone book. Look specifically for Medicaid assistance. You should find a local or toll-free number.

Elderly people who receive Medicare may also be eligible for Medicaid, depending on income level. This is a great help to many people, but too many people are often not aware that they are eligible for both services. If you think this may apply to you, contact your local government's office that provides services to the aged (the phone book will probably help here as well). It is a good idea to get involved with a social worker at these agencies because they are aware of all the services in your area that may be helpful.

Eight

When Things Don't Go Right
Complications, Sick Days, and Problem Solving

Y ou may have noticed that I haven't discussed complications yet. I have a reason for this. I do not believe that patients should be threatened and told things like "unless you do what I tell you terrible things are going to happen to you." Threatening people seldom works. How can you trust someone when he or she threatens you with losing your leg or even your life? How does it help if you are told to follow orders or else? Well, don't worry, I won't threaten you, but you do need important information about complications, so you know why they occur and how to deal with them.

You can do everything you are supposed to and still develop complications. If you don't know what the symptoms are or what they can mean, you may not even recognize a growing complication, so it is very important that you learn as much as you can about this subject. The symptom may not even seem very serious. Remember, nothing that happens to a person with diabetes should be ignored. You can't ignore or wish your problems away. So, if you start developing the symptoms of a complication, your first step is to check with your health care provider. Your problem may be something completely unrelated to your diabetes;

a simple problem that can be treated, cured, and forgotten. Don't let the small problems turn into big ones.

WHY DO PEOPLE WITH DIABETES GET COMPLICATIONS?

Here's an exercise that I love, and it really helps people understand the inner workings of diabetes. It is one of the best tools I use, and I learned it from Dr. Frank Vinicor at the Centers for Disease Control and Prevention. He is a great friend, a wonderful doctor, and an inspiring teacher. You will need a friend or loved one for this exercise.

That's what diabetes is, how it feels, and how your blood sugar levels affect how you feel. I hope you now have an idea of why complications occur, without all the

The Exercise

Instructions: Sit in a comfortable chair with your eyes closed and have a person you trust read the paragraph below to you. It should be read slowly and clearly. Listen to every word and think about what is being said.

Sit comfortably and close your eyes. Just listen to what I say. I want you to think about the blood running through your body. Think about it as if it was nice, cool, spring water. Think about the cool refreshing feel of it going through your body and running around free and easy and smooth and cool. It feels so cool going all about, and it rinses everything clean and clear and comfortable. It goes through just as smoothly as it goes down a nice spring in a green meadow and just feels wonderful. That's what it feels like when your blood sugar is normal and when your blood just goes its merry way all around your body. It goes through the blood vessels of your eyes, and your vision is clear and crisp. It goes through your heart and head and all the blood vessels of your body. Your heart and vessels don't have to work too hard, and they feel the fluid going through easily and smoothly and without effort. You feel cool, comfortable, and not tired. You feel refreshed and relaxed.

It goes to your kidneys and washes out all the impurities and stuff that it's supposed to. It just makes you feel alert and awake, and you are full of energy and vitality. It feels good, and so do you.

Now think about your blood getting thicker. Your blood sugar is up, and the fluid is now about the consistency of maple syrup. It is thick and gooey and having trouble getting around very quickly. It slows down, and the body has to work harder to get it moving. It gets into the fluid behind your eyes, and now you really can't see so clearly. Things are a little blurry. It goes to your blood vessels, and the heart has to work harder to get it pumped around, so your blood pressure goes up. Sometimes you even have headaches or feel it throbbing in your arteries. It goes through your kidneys, and they have to work harder to get it pumped out. The stuff that needs to be carried away is thicker, and your kidneys work harder and harder. Your body is working harder, and you feel more tired. It may be hard work just getting though the day.

The nerves going to your legs get coated with this sticky stuff, and the impulses don't get down to your feet as easily, so you may feel a tingling or pain in your feet and toes. Your feet may feel numb at times, and you may not feel things that you step on. Your body has to work harder to treat or heal infections, and the bacteria have a sweet place to grow now, so you are more prone to infections. This is rough stuff.

(Continued)

> Now, think about taking control and lowering your blood sugars. The thick, sticky stuff starts getting thinner and thinner. It starts moving quickly and easily through your body and clears away all that junk the sticky, sugary stuff left behind. Your heart is not beating so loudly, and your blood pressure is lower. Your eyes are getting clearer, and you feel more alert and comfortable. Your blood is thinner. It is now moving quickly, smoothly, and coolly though your body, and you feel better, lighter, and brighter. You feel good and comfortable. Now, open your eyes.

technical medical jargon, which I will give you next. Does it make it simpler to understand now that you have been through this exercise? If you did not do it, please try it.

Before you go crazy and start thinking of all the things that can go wrong with you, I would like to share some important facts with you that will make you feel better. In the early 1990s, three major studies were done on type 1 and type 2 diabetes that forever changed the way we care for people with diabetes. They were called the DCCT (or Diabetes Control and Complications Trial), the Kumamoto Study, and the United Kingdom Prospective Diabetes Study. These studies showed that tight control could prevent or delay the complications of diabetes.

From these studies, we learned that keeping your blood sugar close to normal levels (between 70 and 99 mg/dl) can reduce your risk of blindness by about 69–76%, your risk of heart attacks by 50%, your risk of kidney disease by 54–70%, and your risk of foot problems by 60%. Think about what these numbers mean. If

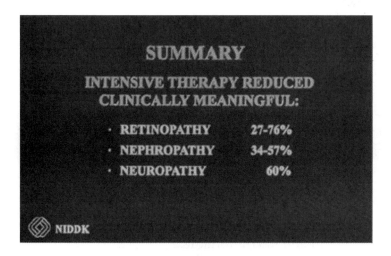

you take care of your diabetes and keep your blood sugars as close to normal as possible, you have a 76% lower chance of becoming blind. Isn't that exciting? You actually have the power to affect your future health by monitoring and managing your blood sugar levels now. These odds are in your favor, and you'd be foolish not to take advantage of them. If someone gave you a lottery ticket and said that you have a 76% chance of winning, wouldn't you take those odds?

But the reality is that complications do occur, and you need to know about them so you can recognize that something is happening and do something about it immediately. Any delay in treatment can be dangerous. Most often, serious complications arise because a patient does not know about complications, their causes, how to prevent them, and how to treat them.

So, let's look at some of the things that can go wrong and that need to be dealt with quickly. These are the short-term or emergency complications. They sometimes occur in people with type 2 diabetes and are often seen in people with type 1 diabetes.

HYPERGLYCEMIA: EXTREMELY HIGH BLOOD SUGARS

So you went to the wedding and ate everything in sight, and now you are feeling rotten. You test and see that your blood sugar is over 300 mg/dl, which is extremely high. You've got **hyperglycemia.** The symptoms of hyperglycemia are simple. They're about the same as how you feel after eating a huge Thanksgiving dinner.

If you have hyperglycemia, you'll feel:

- lethargic (tired and having difficulty moving around)
- very warm and uncomfortable
- warm, dry skin
- very thirsty
- bloated
- blurred vision

Hyperglycemia may also occur when you have an infection or have not taken your medication. Most often, hyperglycemia is treated with careful administration of insulin. There are very specific reasons why your blood sugar goes to hyperglycemic levels.

1. Your meal plan is not working for your blood sugar goals.
2. Your medications need to be adjusted.
3. You need to exercise more.
4. You have an infection.
5. You are going through a major stressful time in your life.

If your blood sugar is above 250 mg/dl, you need to check your urine for ketones with ketone strips. Purchase a bottle of ketone test strips and keep them in your home for these circumstances or on any occasion when your blood sugars are high and hard to manage. It amazes me how many people with diabetes have never heard about ketones or ketone testing. This is an important part of diabetes self-care, and everyone with diabetes should know about ketones and how to test for them.

How to Test for Ketones and Why

Take the test strip out of the bottle; close the bottle securely to keep moisture out. Dip the strip into a sample of your urine and watch the pad at the end change color. Compare the color on the ketone strip to the color chart on the outside of the bottle. This will tell you if you are negative for ketones or have a small, moderate, or large amount of ketones in your urine.

If ketones are absent, low, or moderate, wait two hours and check again. If you have high amounts, you should contact your doctor immediately or go to the emergency room. It is very unusual for a person with type 2 diabetes to have ketones in his or her urine, but that doesn't mean that you shouldn't check. If left untreated, high ketone levels can lead to what we call diabetic ketoacidosis. When your body has too much sugar and not enough insulin to help it burn the sugar, your body starts burning fat. Ketones are an acidic byproduct that is created when your body burns fat, and they can upset your body's natural chemistry and poison you. This is an emergency situation and can lead to what was often called a diabetic coma. It is serious and can be fatal, so be sure to seek help immediately.

Hyperosmolar Hyperglycemic Nonketotic Syndrome

There is a serious condition called hyperosmolar hyperglycemic nonketotic syndrome. It is frequently seen in older people with type 2 diabetes, but can arise in anyone with diabetes. People normally get hyperosmolar hyperglycemic nonketotic syndrome if they have been ill or have an infection.

If you have this syndrome, your blood sugar levels will rise, and your body will try to get rid of the excess sugar by passing it into your urine. You make lots of urine at first, and you have to go to the bathroom more often. Later you may not have to go to the bathroom as often, and your urine becomes very dark. Also, you may be very thirsty. Even if you are not thirsty, you need to drink liquids. If you don't drink enough liquids at this point, you can get dehydrated. If these conditions continue, severe dehydration will lead to seizures, coma, and eventually death. Hyperosmolar hyperglycemic nonketotic syndrome may take days or even weeks to develop.

The Warning Signs of Hyperosmolar Hyperglycemic Nonketotic Syndrome

- Blood sugar level over 600 mg/dl
- Dry, parched mouth
- Extreme thirst (but this may slowly disappear)
- Warm, dry skin that does not sweat
- High fever (over 101 degrees Fahrenheit)
- Sleepiness or confusion
- Loss of vision
- Hallucinations (seeing or hearing things that are not there)
- Weakness on one side of the body

If you have any of these symptoms, call someone on your health care team.

HYPOGLYCEMIA: EXTREMELY LOW BLOOD SUGAR

Because normal blood sugar levels are 70–99 mg/dl, anything below that could be considered low blood sugar. Most people consider low blood sugars to be anything below 70 mg/dl. We call this condition **hypoglycemia.** Think about how you feel when you skip meals; these are often the feelings that come from having low blood sugars. Even people who don't have diabetes can have reactions to low blood sugar. They may have a cold sweat or the shakes. Some people have personality changes and snap at people or get nasty, and they don't even have diabetes. Hypoglycemia is a serious issue and should be treated when it occurs.

I have seen all kinds of responses to hypoglycemia. Some people become confused and nasty, others are unable to talk and start shaking, and some even develop blurry vision and terrible headaches. Sometimes, hypoglycemia shows itself as a feeling of lightheadedness or tremors. Then, there's the opposite: I once had a patient who got so violent when he had hypoglycemia that he threw a television down the hall. I can always tell when my husband is low because he starts getting snippy. I tell him that he is low and should eat something. I like to believe that hypoglycemia makes him nasty sometimes. See, now you have another excuse to give your spouse when you are misbehaving. All joking aside, it is important that you learn how hypoglycemia affects you. I always tell my patients that the best way to identify hypoglycemia is to check your blood sugar when you feel funny.

People with diabetes must carry some kind of quick glucose source with them to prevent hypoglycemia. There are all kinds of simple solutions available. Glucose tablets are made specifically for people with diabetes, and three tablets

Foods with 15 Grams of Carbohydrate

1/2 cup apple juice	6 saltine crackers
1/2 cup regular soda	1/2 cup frozen yogurt
1 Popsicle	1 cup Gatorade
5 Lifesavers	1/4 cup sherbet
1 slice dry toast	1/2 cup regular Jell-O
1/2 cup cooked cereal	1 cup fat-free yogurt

will give you the 15 grams of carbohydrate you need to take immediately. Some people carry Lifesavers or hard candy as their source of 15 grams of carbohydrate. This is called the rule of 15. Take 15 grams of carbohydrate, wait 15 minutes, and test your blood sugar again. If your blood sugar is still low, take another 15 grams of carbohydrate. Wait 15 more minutes and test again. If it is still low, call your doctor. For someone who has type 1 diabetes, hypoglycemia must be treated quickly, before he or she falls unconscious. This can be fatal and is a medical emergency.

SICK DAYS

Everybody gets sick sometimes. If you have diabetes, though, a cold or flu can be serious. Make sure that you get a flu shot every year and a pneumonia shot once every 10 years. If you are sick and are vomiting or have diarrhea, you are losing fluids and glucose from your body. If you are ill, you need to keep your body hydrated. If you cannot keep fluid down at all (by vomiting it up or through diarrhea), you may require intravenous fluids (these are given to you through a tube), which requires a visit to the emergency room or your doctor's office. Here are some basic rules to follow when you are sick:

1. Test your blood sugar every four hours. Test your urine for ketones.
2. Drink at least 8 ounces of calorie-free fluid, preferably water, every hour while you are awake.
3. If you cannot keep any fluids or food down, notify your doctor so you can get medications to stop the vomiting.

Smoking

There is another special consideration that needs to be front and center. Any patient with diabetes who smokes needs to quit. I cannot stress enough how dangerous this is and what you would be doing to your chances of living a longer, healthier life if you decide that smoking is more important than quitting. I know how hard it is to give up smoking because I have been teaching people how to quit smoking for years. Some people say that smoking is harder to give up than a cocaine addiction. I don't know about that, but I do know people who have tried quitting for years or who have stopped smoking for decades and then gone back. This is frustrating and frightening, and people need all of the help they can get. There are wonderful programs all over the country that may help you, such as hypnotism, medications, and group therapy sessions. Look around, and you will find help.

Talk to your doctor about nicotine patches, gum, and pills. These are often pretty successful programs that help people to quit smoking. Also, keep an eye out for the new medications that are now in scientific trials and should be released in the near future. However, none of these aids will help if you are not determined to quit. That decision is yours and yours alone. No treats or rewards, begging, or bribes from your friends, family, or loved ones will help. The only thing that stops a person from smoking is a person who wants to quit.

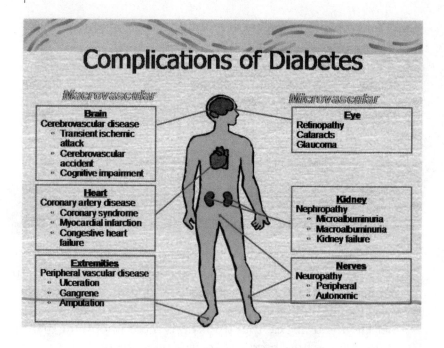

4. Insulin and most oral medications should be taken as normal, but your dosages may need to be adjusted for your blood sugar levels.
5. Eat soft foods or drink fluids with glucose to keep away hypoglycemia, if you can't keep down regular, solid foods.

CARDIAC COMPLICATIONS

People with diabetes have a four times greater chance of developing heart disease. Here are some of the different types of cardiac complications that we are concerned with:

- coronary artery disease
- peripheral arterial disease
- coronary syndrome

- myocardial infarction (heart attack)
- congestive heart failure

These are some of the killer problems that can arise, but you've probably also heard about other heart and circulatory issues, such as bypass surgeries and strokes. If your blood doesn't flow properly to your legs and feet (a condition called peripheral arterial disease), then you may be at greater risk of a heart attack or stroke. So you need to consider all of those blood vessels and arteries, too, and try to keep them healthy. Because you're at an increased danger of developing heart and circulatory problems, you need to look after more than just your blood sugars. Let's talk about the ABCs of diabetes self-care.

A1C

The recommended goal is to keep your A1C levels below 7%. This is the standard of care that the American Diabetes Association sets for people who have already been diagnosed with diabetes. The new goal for people with diabetes has been to get A1C levels as close to 6% as possible without serious side effects. I've already harped about this enough, so you should know by now that keeping your blood sugar levels down can really help you over the long term.

Blood Pressure

You should keep an eye on your blood pressure, and the recommended goal is below 130/80 mmHg. Keeping your blood pressure at this level will help protect your heart and your kidneys from future damage. Remember that the higher your blood pressure, the harder your heart is working and the more stress is being put on your kidneys. Things that work harder wear out faster, so keep your blood pressure as close to normal as possible.

Cholesterol

Your cholesterol numbers tell you the amount of fat in your blood. Remember that there are different kinds of cholesterol, both good and bad.

The good cholesterol is HDL, and it stands for high-density lipoprotein. I remember it by **H** for **Healthy.** HDL is the good stuff that keeps your blood vessels lubricated and prevents plaque and clots from sticking to the walls of your blood vessels, leading to clogged or hardened arteries. The best way to raise your HDL is through regular exercise and movement. Your HDL should be above 40 if you are a man and above 50 if you are a woman.

The cholesterol that clogs your blood vessels and puts you at risk for strokes and heart attack is LDL, which stands for low-density lipoprotein. Remember that LDL choles-terol is **Lousy.** The American Heart Association recom-mends keeping your LDL below 100, but we are now aim-ing for 70. You can start lowering your LDL cholesterol level by cutting saturated fats and trans fats from your diet.

Triglycerides are another kind of fat in your blood, and they also raise your risks of heart disease. You need to keep your triglycerides below 150.

You'll also get a number called your total cholesterol, which is a general rating of the total amount of cholesterol in your blood. You won't get your total cholesterol number by adding your HDL and LDL cholesterol together.

Your doctor may put you on medications, such as statins, to help you keep healthy lipid (fat) levels. There is a whole new movement that aims to aggressively treat blood

Aspirin Can Help Keep Your Heart Healthy

I know I've mentioned this in chapter 2, but it's worth discussing again. Many scientific studies have shown that taking a low dose of aspirin (81 mg) every day can help lower your risk of heart attacks and strokes. No one is exactly sure why this is true, but it likely has something to do with the fact that aspirin keeps your blood from clumping together. When your blood clumps together, it can block your blood vessels and cause a heart attack or stroke.

Before you rush out to buy that bottle of aspirin, though, please discuss it with your health care providers. Aspirin is not the right choice for everyone. People can have allergic reactions to aspirin or other preexisting conditions could react badly to the aspirin. Remember, it's always better to be safe than sorry, so check with your doctor first.

fat levels, too, in order to prevent their associated complications before they can occur.

RETINOPATHY

Diabetic retinopathy is a term that describes several types of changes that affect the retina of the eye. It can be mild or severe and may even cause blindness. Because diabetes is the major cause of blindness in the U.S., retinopathy is not something to take lightly. If diagnosed early, it can be treated and blindness can be prevented.

You need to get annual eye examinations from an eye doctor who specializes in the diseases and problems of the eye. When you first visit the ophthalmologist, you should

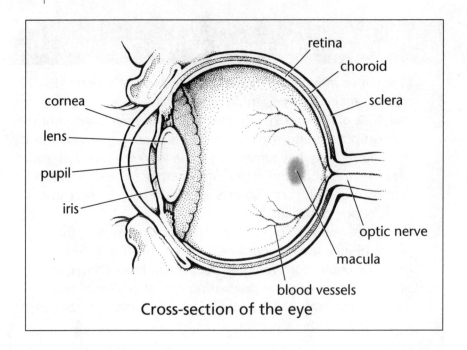

Cross-section of the eye

have a picture taken of your retina. This is called a baseline photo and will show the status of your retina. Even more, having this photo taken now will give you something to compare to later on, because then you can see if the condition of your retina has changed much over time. This is very important. Please remember that with good management of your blood sugar levels, you can dramatically reduce the chances of developing retinopathy.

Retinopathy often develops because of hemorrhages in the small blood vessels in the retina. Each hemorrhage causes a blind spot, and the more hemorrhages you have, the less vision you have. We can deal with these small hemorrhages and prevent them from causing more damage by using laser surgery. You may have heard people saying that they have had several "burns" to their eye. The laser is used to seal the damaged blood vessel by burning it. This stops the bleeding and keeps it from bleeding again. There is also an experimental medication being studied that may reduce the vision loss from retinopathy.

NEUROPATHY

Dr. Fran Kaufman, past president of the American Diabetes Association, describes neuropathy as "an attack on the information highway." **Neuropathy** means nerve damage. Your nerves keep your brain in contact with the rest of your body and control many of the body's necessary functions, such as moving your limbs and keeping your heart beating. When you have diabetes, the sugar in your blood attaches to the proteins in your nerve fibers and to the insulation that surrounds them. This damages your nerves, and they cannot transmit the information that makes your body work smoothly. Nerve damage can be painful and is sometimes difficult to manage.

Neuropathy is the most common of all diabetes complications. About half of all people with diabetes eventually develop some kind of nerve damage. Neuropathy can be very painful, and sometimes patients are grateful when the pain goes away. Sadly, that is not always a great thing because when the pain stops, it may be an indication that the nerves are dead. This can lead to lack of circulation. When your circulation is impaired, your wounds will not heal well and infections can become a major health hazard. The final and worst complication of neuropathy is amputation, because the limb has suffered from infections and tissue death due to poor circulation. Amputations are still occurring too frequently. Only aggressive treatment of any wound or infection can prevent these terrible consequences. Too many people have a memory of a family member or friend who lost a limb because of insufficient diabetes care. Remember, you can reduce your chances of developing neuropathy by carefully managing your blood sugar levels.

Foot Problems

When you lose sensation in your feet due to neuropathy, you cannot feel a bruise or wound. Left untreated, these small injuries can turn into huge problems. That's why daily foot inspections and foot care are so important. Proper shoes are absolutely necessary. When you think of saving money, don't do it by buying cheap or tight shoes. A few extra dollars spent on the right shoes can save your feet and legs. I'm going to give you a ton of great tips for proper foot care, so you can make sure the terrible effects of neuropathy don't get in the way of a healthy, happy life.

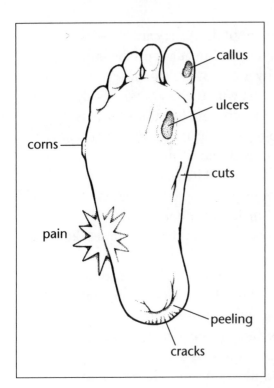

Get Your Doctor to Check Your Feet

The most important thing I can tell you is to take off your shoes and socks each time you go to your doctor's office. Data show that physicians sometimes forget to examine your feet unless you remind them, and I do not want you to miss this important part of proper diabetes care.

Examine Your Feet Daily

Even if you have no pains or tingling in your feet, you need to inspect them visually. Wash your feet each day and carefully inspect them. It's amazing what people accidentally step on. People have walked into my classes with sharp objects stuck in their feet, like pins and staples. They stepped on these things and because of nerve damage never knew that they were there. Make sure that you check between your toes and carefully clean and dry them. When you are caring for and drying your feet, avoid using powders, such as talcum powder, because when powder combines with water, little beads can form between the toes and cause irritations that become open sores.

You should never walk around barefoot, especially outside. You cannot imagine how much damage you can do to

I don't know about you, but I have trouble seeing the entire bottom of my foot. If you have the same problem as me, I suggest that you buy a mirror with a long handle. If you have one of these, you won't have to twist yourself into a pretzel to inspect the bottoms of your feet. Look for any splits in the skin on the bottom of your feet or between your toes. Look for red or dark spots that have not been there before. When you press on the bottom of your foot, does the redness go away and return immediately? Is the foot swollen or tender? These may be signs of infection, so contact your doctor for a professional inspection.

There is an instrument that we use to test for loss of feeling. It is called a monofilament. We use size 5.07, and you can try this at home with a piece of stiff fishing line. When we use this test, we stick the foot in many places: on the bottom of your toes, on the soles of your feet below the toes, and on your heels. You should feel the touch of the monofilament every time. If you do not, then you may be losing sensation and should talk to your doctor.

your feet just walking on the beach barefoot, for example. Remember that shells and coral are organic material and harbor bacteria. I recommend buying waterproof shoes to wear on the beach and in the water, even in pools. Pool floors are often rough, and you can stub your toe or cut your foot on the bottom.

Keep Your Feet Lubricated

Cream your feet with a good lubricating cream and keep them soft and free of calluses. You should never ever cut calluses with a razor or blade of any kind. This is very dangerous. If you're losing sensation, you may cut too deep and open yourself to the risks of infection. If at all possible, go to a podiatrist for regular foot care. Medicare will pay for a podiatrist visit every nine weeks and more often if you have neuropathy or any documented foot problems. Most insurance companies will pay for frequent visits. Podiatrists are often familiar with diabetes and will give you sound advice and good treatments. They are excellent professionals but are unfortunately often overlooked as a part of anyone's diabetes support team. You should try to include one in your support group.

Get Circulation in Your Feet

Diabetes is enough of a problem; don't make the circulation to your feet any worse than it has to be. When you are sitting around, put your feet up. Don't sit with your legs crossed. If you are on a long airplane flight, get up and walk around every hour. Wear comfortable socks that fit properly and never wear anything tight around your legs. I know some elderly women who wear knee highs instead of pantyhose. There are tight, deep marks on their legs when they remove them. This is not a safe practice. So do your-

There is a lot of discussion about whether people with diabetes should have pedicures. The most important thing is for you to avoid infection. If you really want pedicures, make sure you bring your own nail clippers and scissors and make sure that everything the manicurist uses is used on only you, including the foot tub. You do not want to catch a fungal infection from another client. You might want to discuss pedicures with your doctor or diabetes educator.

self a favor and get comfortable. Keep that blood flowing through your feet.

NEPHROPATHY

Nephropathy is kidney damage. When you have diabetes, your kidneys are working harder to rid your body of extra sugar in your blood. This constant hard work eventually damages them. They get worn out. We check for kidney damage by testing your urine for **microalbuminuria,** which means that there is protein in your urine. It is one of the first signs of problems with the kidneys. If this problem is left unchecked, the kidneys can be damaged so badly that they stop functioning. When nephropathy goes untreated, you can wind up on dialysis, which is when your blood is filtered through a machine to clean it instead of through your kidneys. Ultimately, nephropathy can lead to kidney failure, which is fatal.

You should be very careful to tell every doctor you see that you have diabetes. There are medications that can damage your kidneys, so by telling your doctors about your diabetes, you can prevent this terrible mistake from ever happening. Your doctor may put you on a medication called an ACE inhibitor to protect your kidneys from future damage.

CONCLUSIONS

These are the complications of diabetes. They sound scary, and they are, but you should take home the message that with proper care and management of your blood sugars, blood pressure, and cholesterol, you can delay or prevent them from ever happening. I didn't write this section to scare you, but to make you think about the important things that can happen to people with diabetes. Remember, the percentages are in your favor. Take care of yourself, and it is very likely that you can avoid complications.

Keeping Yourself Motivated

We have now talked about all of the steps necessary to get you involved and informed in taking care of your diabetes. I hope at this point that you have made decisions about what you are willing to do to take care of yourself. If you have, that's great, but there will always be moments when you'll wonder how you will be able to go on. I hope that all the time we've spent together has helped you get excited and motivated to take the next steps in caring for yourself. Still, no matter what I say, somewhere in the far back of your mind there may be some doubts. You may be thinking something like, "Well, Ginger's really into this diabetes stuff and that's great, but she is just one person and doesn't have diabetes like me." I understand this, and I know that you can move past these doubts. Remember, I've been treating people with diabetes for decades.

I want to share more than my excitement about helping people with diabetes. I want to share with you the people who have turned me on to diabetes care, got me started on this wonderful path, kept me going when diabetes seemed like it was too much to overcome, and made my job joyful. Everything I know about diabetes has come from my patients and my colleagues who teach them. Treating and caring for people with diabetes is a two-way street. I have learned from other educators as they have learned from me in conferences, meetings, seminars, and in halls with thousands of diabetes educators and health care professionals. A lot of the best learning came from hours spent in the clinic. One of the best learning experiences of my life was when I served as President of the American Association of Diabetes Educators. I am so honored to have been among the brightest, most caring people in the world, and sometimes I wondered what I had done to be considered to stand among such brilliant people.

But it is the people with diabetes, and the people who live with them, who are the true teachers, guides, and mentors of the diabetes world. They will motivate you and inspire you and will be there to support you when you need a hand or a shoulder to cry on. It is so important to know that you don't have to tackle the difficulty of living with a chronic disease alone. I hope this book can help you take the road toward a very long, healthy, happy life. To thank you and to help you, I'm giving you three small gifts to keep you motivated through those rough spots.

MY FIRST GIFT: WORDS OF WISDOM

Here is my first gift: I am giving you words of wisdom from some of the brightest, best minds in the diabetes world. If nothing else I hope it will give you that little extra push to smile your way through diabetes self-care. I want to give you a little bit of hope that you can turn to when it seems like that's the last thing you can imagine having. So I went to the wonderful diabetes educators I know and asked them to send me their words of wisdom. The question was very simple: "If you could give a person with diabetes your favorite piece of advice, what would it be?" Here are their answers.

PAIGE REDDEN MS, RD, CDE

"My advice? Just be happy that it isn't something else. Something you have no control over. Diabetes is in your control. Learn all you can, get a great health care team surrounding you, and don't stand for anything less than knowledgeable, supportive physicians and diabetes educators. Then go take control and be the healthiest you have ever been. Many people have felt it was a blessing—a knocking on the door—that finally woke them up. You are never given more than you can handle!"

KEITH CAMPBELL RPH, FASHP, MBA, CDE

"I have now had diabetes for 57 years. The best advice that I received when I developed diabetes came from my physician and from my father. Both told me that there were many positive aspects of having diabetes and that I would learn a lot about how the body works. I could eat healthy meals, take my insulin, manage my blood sugars, and, as Patti Labelle says, 'I have diabetes, diabetes does not have me.' They also pointed out that I would have a life challenge to overcome. If I had a positive attitude and took charge of my diabetes, I would live a near-normal and great life. Their advice proved to be true, and as I look back, having diabetes has been more of a blessing to me than a burden."

CAROLÉ MENSING RN, MA, CDE

"You and I are partners in this diabetes journey. My role is to help you be better at managing diabetes than I am or could ever be! Diabetes education makes a difference!"

GARY ARSHAM MD, PhD

"What I would share with a person with diabetes is the importance of informed personal choices, based on that person's personal values and the best information available. The act of conscious and mindful choosing becomes the foundation of our ability to manage diabetes effectively. If you have diabetes, it is also important to recognize the need for balance; that is, taking care of your diabetes while dealing with the other demands in your life. Of course, this is also the main theme of <u>Diabetes: A Guide to Living Well, 4th Edition.</u>"

WENDY DREW RN, BSN, CDE

"While striving for your <u>best</u>, there are times when <u>good</u> and <u>better</u> have a place. Make a change that is <u>good</u>, move on to what is <u>better</u>, and you will end up with your <u>best</u>. This is especially helpful as you move through the less-charted waters of diabetes self-management. If you are not sure of the ultimate goal, then you can always move from good to better to best."

JOANNE GALLIVAN MS, RD, NDEP

"My piece of advice to the person with diabetes is to remember that you are the most important member of the health care team. Although the professionals on the health care team bring years of experience and lots of expertise, the most important member is you."

HOPE WARSHAW MMSC, RD, CDE

"First, try to find a provider and diabetes educator with whom you can form a partnership. You don't have to work with providers or educators who make unrealistic demands. Find people who want to understand you, your needs, and your lifestyle—people who want to help you fit diabetes into your life, not the opposite. Second, you will have your good days and not-so-good days, whether that applies to blood sugar control or how you feel, so try not to judge yourself harshly and chastise yourself. Do use all of the experiences you encounter to gain insight and better understanding of how to best manage your diabetes."

MARY BETH FISHER APRN, BC, CDE

"First, you are a person. Included in your journey, as a unique being, is the challenge of living with diabetes. The action is indeed that: <u>living</u> with diabetes. The hope is to <u>live</u> well. Keep an open mind. Be informed. Make healthy choices. Ask for help. Use help when it is offered. Perfection is not required or expected. Take time for personal retreats for rejuvenation and 're-creation' (not just recreation). When there is a bump in the road, deal with it and move on. You are important. Believe it."

JERRY MEECE RPH, FACA, CDE

"I think the most important thing you need to remember is that you are the one in charge of your care. Understand that 95% of the success of controlling your diabetes is up to you and only 5% is up to all the professionals who support you with advice and care. We can show you how and when and even tell you why you need to do certain things, but we can't inject for you, exercise for you, or decide what and how much you eat day in and day out. The second-most important thing is to have patience. We'll work together, and you'll learn about <u>your</u> diabetes much like the way you eat an apple, one bite at a time. One day, just like you would have eaten the whole apple, you will have a large amount of knowledge about what works for you and that in itself will make your life easier."

JOY PAPE RN, BSN, CDE, WOCN, CFCN

"No doubt about it, it takes work to manage your diabetes. It takes work to accomplish anything that's worth something in this world. Always remember this: it's a lot easier to prevent the complications of diabetes than to live with them."

MARCIA DRAHIEM RN, CDE

"No person with diabetes can 'live perfectly enough' to have all of his or her blood sugar tests fall within the recommended ranges. Please lift this burden from your shoulders. As much as possible, do your best. Recognize that sometimes 'life happens.' Your blood sugar tests do not give you 'good' or 'bad' numbers. They are rather like numbers on a fuel gauge, speedometer, and compass that let you know how well and quickly your body is utilizing its fuel and the direction needed to best control your blood sugars."

HELEN AMUNDSON RN, CDE

"Thank you for the opportunity to pass on the pearls of wisdom that I tell my patients. I tell them to remember that they are the captain of the ship and we are their crew. They are in charge of their diabetes, and it is our job to help them find the tools to help them get to where they want to be with their diabetes."

BRENDA A. BROUSSARD RD, MPH, MBA, BC-ADM, CDE

"Here are some thoughts:

- "Learn all you can about how your body responds to food, activity, and medicines. You can balance your diabetes. Learn more. Talk with your doctor and your certified diabetes educator—coaches who help you balance your diabetes and daily life.
- "Become a diabetes advocate. Share your story about the challenges and lessons of life with diabetes. Share your story with your family, friends, elected officials—especially Congress, so that there is support for you and others with diabetes and that there are enough funds for diabetes research, treatment, and self-care education.
- "To get the most out of your health care visits: write down your concerns and questions, share your food diary, bring your blood glucose logbook or meter (with memory), and bring your activity log to your health care providers.
- "Studies show that very happy people spend at least 10 minutes each day doing what they thoroughly enjoy.
- "Studies show that very happy people find the gift in every experience."

MARY M. AUSTIN MA, RD, CDE

"Along with your diagnosis of diabetes, which I am sure you are a bit apprehensive about, you have the unique opportunity to take 'stock' of your current lifestyle. Up to this point you may not have given your health or lifestyle much thought. How you choose to live your life from this day forward will impact your future. To live successfully with diabetes means that you will need to adopt some lifestyle changes. Most patients say 'eating right' and 'getting active' are the most challenging. I suggest to my patients that they buy a small notebook (anything spiral bound will do) and, every day for about a week or so, write down the following:

- all food and beverages consumed and the time of day
- any physical activity (biking, walking, swimming, etc.) and time spent doing that activity

"After a week or so, go back and look at what you have recorded and ask yourself the following questions:

- What is my eating pattern? Do I eat one meal a day?
- What is my schedule of eating? Do I eat at consistent times of day or haphazard?
- Am I eating fresh fruits, vegetables, and whole grains each day? How much?
- What processed, prepared foods am I eating?
- How many times a week do I eat away from home?
- How much physical activity do I get each day? Some? None?

"The answers to these questions should give you a clue as to where you can start to make some lifestyle changes to improve your health and successfully manage your diabetes. You decide what you would like to accomplish first, and I will help you. Even small changes, consistently maintained over time, can make a big difference! Patients have told me that since their diagnosis of diabetes, they are living healthier than ever before. You can, too!"

GERALYN SPOLLETT RN, C-ANP, CDE

"Although we talk about blood glucose control, there are many more components involved in achieving this than just exercise, food, and insulin. We know that insulin works to lower glucose levels, but our wonderful bodies make many more hormones that work in ways that raise glucose levels by promoting the release of stored glucose in places such as the liver and the muscle. These hormones work on 'automatic pilot'; in other words, we have limited control over them. Despite our best efforts to keep everything in balance, there are times when glucose levels, responding to these 'other' hormones, will be higher than anticipated. Don't beat yourself up over this! Do what you can to lower the glucose level and then move on, you have a life to live.

"When patients tell me that they are very tired and it seems that their glucose levels and A1C are relatively stable, I ask them probing questions to rule out sleep apnea. My advice is this: if you are falling asleep during the day, wake up each morning with a dry throat and mouth, or your spouse complains that the snoring or jerking motions you make keep waking him or her, then tell your care provider about these problems because you may have sleep apnea. A simple test can check you for this condition, which is becoming increasingly more common in people with diabetes, both men and women. Sleep apnea can add stress to your heart and increase insulin resistance. Treatment will help you sleep better and healthier."

CHRISTY L. PARKIN MSN, RN, CDE

"Don't wait until tomorrow to start making positive changes in your life. Start today. Everything that you are being advised to do—eating right, losing weight, and getting some regular exercise—are changes that just about everyone should be making, even if they don't have diabetes. Although you won't feel the physical benefits of these changes for at least a couple of weeks, you will immediately feel the positive benefits of taking control of your life. Every day that you wake up and make a conscious decision to live a healthier life, and then follow through, is a successful day. Eventually you will reap more tangible benefits from your actions. Having diabetes is no blessing, but it does provide an opportunity to significantly improve your physical, mental, and spiritual health. It's your choice as to whether to act upon this opportunity. You've got nothing to lose and everything to gain."

TERESA L. PEARSON MS, RN, CDE

"Diabetes can be overwhelming. Take it in small steps and ask for help. There are a lot of people out there who are more than willing to help you. View your relationship with your health care team as a partnership, where you are the expert in your diabetes. Your plan on how you will manage your diabetes will have been developed in collaboration with your diabetes care team. It is important for you to know all of the facets of diabetes and your life. Know diabetes, know yourself, know how you are doing, know when to ask for help, know your diabetes care team, know what to expect of your diabetes care team, and know who you can rely on for support. Knowledge is power. It will help you stay in control of your diabetes. Recognize that diabetes is a part of who you are but not all of who you are."

MY SECOND GIFT: REAL-LIFE EXPERIENCES

I hope the theme of these letters—how you need to be in charge and work with your team—comes through loud and clear. I did not prompt these experts or tell them the subject for their comments. It is amazing how the same thought appeared over and over again. Maybe the 20,000 diabetes educators out there have come to the same conclusion because it really is true and really makes sense.

My second gift to you is a real-life story about two wonderful people. I would like to share one of my favorite stories about a patient. I have published it before, and it was on the website DiabetesinControl.com, but it is such a great look at the contradictions that arise when you have diabetes that I want to share it with you. This story will give you a good

opportunity to look at the choices people make and how
they can change your life.

This is the story about two women, whom I shall call
Tara and Sara. I met them recently in Florida, and they
are originally from New York, just as I am. They are very
interesting, bright, articulate women and represent two
of the types of people with diabetes that I have taught
for most of my career.

Both are retired, professional women in their late
sixties and are college educated. Both are still married
to very pleasant, caring men and have children and
grandchildren. They happen to be sisters-in-law. Both
have a comfortable life that they have earned and
deserve. Both are charming and lots of fun. Both have
type 2 diabetes.

Tara is very concerned about her diabetes and is
determined to be in the best condition and heath status possible for the rest of her life. I met her while she
was exercising at the swimming pool. She walks two
to five miles every day, faithfully takes her insulin, and
checks her blood sugar four times a day. She gets
upset with peaks and valleys and tries to keep her
blood sugar levels as close to normal as possible. She
is a partner with her endocrinologist—who is two and
a half hours away by car—and asks and reads about
everything that has to do with diabetes. She will
attend any class or support group available. Lest you
think that she is a "professional diabetic patient," she
also has a very rich, full life. She and her husband are
also wonderful dancers. Tara isn't quite a saint,
though; she likes to eat rich desserts at dances, and
she thinks I don't notice. Now that we are friends, she
has included me in her team. It is a pleasure.

Sara introduced herself to me as the "other type of diabetic." She was rather overweight and did not exercise at all. She tested her blood when she remembered to and was embarrassed to tell me, even though I never asked her to. At the time, she told me that she was not a "real diabetic" because she didn't take insulin. She said that she was not prepared to be a diabetic and had no real problems or complications with it. *Yet.* I asked her if she had ever been to a class or course on diabetes or been under the care of a diabetes educator. She took a class once a long time ago. She said that it was not very interesting, that she really couldn't get into it, and that she couldn't even remember the name of the educator. Her doctor made her go, but it really did not matter to her. After all, she was the "other kind of diabetic."

Does this sound familiar? It made me sad to think of this really nice woman walking around in "diabetes limbo." I am concerned that we, as diabetes educators and health care providers, somehow missed the boat with Sara. Somehow we never had or created a teachable moment where suddenly, everything fell into place for Sara. We did not turn her on to her own responsibilities and abilities or motivate her to want to care for herself. Now it was going to be much harder for Sara to get into the habit of taking care of herself.

For many years I believed that if patients did not learn, then I had not taught them correctly. I had failed and was a poor excuse for an educator. It took a long time for me to understand that education is a partnership.

Sara was in denial. She didn't want to be a "diabetic" or to have to deal with it. As a grown woman, she had to make her own decisions and live with the consequences of those decisions. She was not ready to learn, and it took a very long time for her to reach the stage where she accepted that she needed to learn and needed some help. She was not at all interested in seeing the educator I recommended. People need to make their own decisions, and I don't believe you can empower a patient with a club or by holding hostages (a little saying I learned from experts, Bob Anderson and Marti Funnell). Instead, I stuck Tara and her husband on the case of persuading Sara and hoped they would finally get to her. It was the best that I could do.

Recently, I saw Tara again, and she is doing very well. She is on a new insulin regimen and is doing much better with her low blood sugars. She has lost 30 pounds due to moving homes and some family stress, but she has no intention of losing more. She says it is fun to have a few pounds to gain. She looks wonderful and feels good. What about Sara?

I saw Sara recently, and she is a new person. Her doctor put her on a new medication. She has lost a great deal of weight and looks and feels wonderful. She bought a new wardrobe, and now she and Tara are a sight to behold. Good for both of them! Sara decided to take care of herself. Now she is amazed that it took her years to make that choice.

MY THIRD GIFT: WISDOM FROM MY PATIENTS

Here is my third gift to you. It is the best thing I could think of to have this all make sense. I asked three of my patients to answer two questions. First, how did you feel when you found out you had diabetes? Second, if you could give new patients advice about living with diabetes, what would you tell them? These are their letters to you.

Dear Newly Diagnosed Diabetic,

I really had not known too much about diabetes when I was originally diagnosed. My doctor gave me a book to read that made me realize the seriousness of the disease.

I was a bit frightened at the beginning, but the more knowledge I obtained, the more I realized that taking good care of myself, getting a good team of health providers (endocrinologist, podiatrist, ophthalmologist, diabetes educator, and nutritionist), and having a positive attitude would help me lead a normal life and avoid complications.

Most of all, I learned that basically I was the one in charge of doing the right things for myself and my health. The lifestyle of a diabetic—eating properly, exercising, no smoking, weight control, good teeth, and health care—is best for anyone, diabetic or not. It's a healthy lifestyle!

Learn about watching your A1C and ask your doctors to explain and answer any of your questions. Read about what's new. Knowledge truly is power.

Testing my blood glucose and injecting insulin is no big chore. I consider it a good habit, like brushing my teeth a few times a day. It's good for me, so I do what I have to and then get on with my life!

I enjoy my children and grandchildren. My husband and I go dancing with our good friends and travel in this country and abroad. We go out to eat and enjoy swimming, shows, and the movies. I feel well.

Live and laugh. There's so much to enjoy. Life is good!

Sincerely,

Thelma "Timmy" Rabin

This letter was sent to me several years ago and was included in my book for professionals, "Patient Education: You Can Do It!" This letter has so much valuable advice that I just had to share it with you.

Dear Ginger,

As I look back on my own life, it is obvious that education has not influenced my understanding of how the body functions or my management of my health. We are all told that we have to eat a balanced diet and get exercise, but so what? As my lifestyle changed from participating in sports to working in construction to business management, I've been consistently surprised by the health consequences of my lifestyle choices.

As my health problems have become too annoying to ignore, I have gone to the doctor. Without exception, the information received from the doctor was inadequate. He can't be an educator because of time constraints, so I have had to do research, ask questions, and try to ferret out what to do. When my blood pressure was measured at 160/95 and exercise was prescribed, it was a surprise and a revelation to see it drop to 116/68 consistently. When it became unacceptable to feel mean and angry two hours after a meal, a change to a low-carbohydrate, high-protein diet with fruits and vegetables changed everything. I now enjoy a peaceful feeling all day.

When my best friend became pale and almost passed out, it hit me that he was constantly drinking water all day long. So we measured his blood sugar level on a diabetic friend's machine, saw that his numbers were in the high

(continued)

300s, and called you. His blood sugar levels are managed according to a new way of teaching people how the body functions, but without your help and input, this management would have been woefully inadequate.

We go to the doctor for a check-up because we should or because of a crisis. We leave OK or with a prescription. We certainly can't leave the office well educated as to how our lifestyle affects our health. It is very difficult to find information on what to do next. There should be a prescription for meaningful education and follow-up.

The management of one's health should not begin in a crisis, when the damage is already done. Health education should be designed and made available so that more people are reached and then effort should be made to actually change their lifestyle to a healthy one. We should all be educated to react to changes in lifestyle that will damage our health and be able to understand symptoms of problems that require a visit to the doctor.

Sincerely,

Courtland

Dear Newly Diagnosed Diabetic,

I am a 78-year-old man who was diagnosed as a type 2 diabetic eight years ago. This diagnosis was the result of my annual physical exam, the good results of which I always took for granted. Now I had found out news that frightened me to no end. The doctor had advised me to lose weight and to exercise. He also gave me some literature to read, but never mentioned the use of a meter to check my glucose level. I left that office with a feeling of dread.

Visions of strict diets, amputations, and, worst of all, potential blindness filled my mind. I knew that only my wife would be told about my diabetes. I could not bring myself to tell anyone else because it was always difficult to admit to any "weakness" or "deficiencies" on my part.

So, up until two years ago, I suffered through extreme diets (which I continually violated), visited my doctor regularly, and always worried about my feet and eyes. That is, until I met a diabetes educator in the Florida Keys. This lady offered a seminar that realistically allayed my fears, taught me how to obtain and use a glucose meter, and assured me that I could live a normal life, even with my illness.

Like an orchestra conductor, this lady "tapped her baton," answered every question, looked at every "player," and gave us confidence. She assured us that all would be well if we followed the rules. We realized then that education is the main factor for coping with diabetes.

I now face my diabetes with confidence and strength and with the knowledge that "I am the captain of my fate. I am the master of my soul!"

Sincerely,

Morris Weiler

I cannot think of a better way to send you off into the world of diabetes than with Morrie's great advice.

Resources and References

Y ou know about diabetes now, and I hope that you have a good idea about how to keep yourself motivated. Now, the last thing I'm going to give you is some starting points on where to go for additional information. In this chapter, you'll find organizations to contact, websites to visit, and wonderful materials to read. I have decided that people don't often know where to go to find the materials they need, so I am including some starting points right here. There is a list of books from the American Diabetes Association and other sources. There is a list of the websites and phone numbers of companies and organizations that provide patient education, too. I really want you to join the community of people who know what is available to them, so please get out there and get in contact with any of these wonderful associations. Have fun and enjoy the journey!

ASSOCIATIONS AND GOVERNMENT OFFICES

American Association of Diabetes Educators

The AADE is a wonderful association that helps diabetes educators and sets standards for high-quality diabetes self-management education.

Website: www.diabeteseducator.org
Phone: 1-800-338-3633

American Diabetes Association

The American Diabetes Association is the nation's leading nonprofit health organization providing diabetes research, information, and advocacy. Founded in 1940, the American Diabetes Association conducts programs in all 50 states and the District of Columbia, reaching hundreds of communities. The mission of the association is to prevent and cure diabetes and to improve the lives of all people affected by diabetes.

Website: www.diabetes.org
Phone: 1-800-DIABETES

American Dietetic Association

The American Dietetic Association is the nation's largest organization of food and nutrition professionals. It sets the standards of practice for dietitians throughout the U.S. and is constantly identifying ways to improve the nutritional health of the American public.

Website: www.eatright.org
Phone: 1-800-877-1600

Centers for Disease Control and Prevention

The Centers for Disease Control and Prevention, as the sentinel for the health of people in the U.S. and throughout the world, strives to protect people's health and safety, provide reliable health information, and improve health through strong partnerships. They are responsible for translating all of the research on diabetes into the practical care of people with diabetes.

Website: www.cdc.gov
Phone: 1-800-311-3435

Centers for Medicare and Medicaid Services

The mission of the Centers for Medicare and Medicaid Services is to ensure effective, up-to-date health care coverage and to promote quality care for beneficiaries. This government office is responsible for making sure that Medicare and Medicaid pays for the appropriate care for people with diabetes.

Website: http://www.cms.hhs.gov/
Phone: 1-800-633-4227

International Diabetes Federation

The International Diabetes Federation (IDF) is a worldwide alliance of 200 diabetes associations in 158 countries that have come together to enhance the lives of people with diabetes everywhere. For over 50 years, the IDF has been at the forefront of global diabetes advocacy. It is committed to raising global awareness of diabetes, promoting appropriate diabetes care and prevention, and encouraging activities toward finding a cure for the different types of diabetes. It is the mission of IDF to promote diabetes care, prevention, and a cure worldwide.

Website: www.idf.org
E-mail: info@idf.org

Juvenile Diabetes Research Foundation

The Juvenile Diabetes Research Foundation (JDRF) is the leading charitable funding organization and advocate of type 1 diabetes research worldwide. The mission of JDRF is to find a cure for diabetes and its complications through the support of research.

Website: www.jdf.org
Phone: 1-800-533-CURE

National Diabetes Education Program
The National Diabetes Education Program (NDEP) is a federally funded program sponsored by the U.S. Department of Health and Human Services' National Institutes of Health and the Centers for Disease Control and Prevention and includes over 200 partners at the federal, state, and local levels, working together to reduce the morbidity and mortality associated with diabetes. NDEP produces diabetes education guidelines for health care professionals and produces diabetes education materials for people with diabetes. NDEP has the benefit of a huge consortium of partners to rely on as experts when they put this information together. NDEP produces educational materials in over 13 languages.

Website: www.ndep.nih.gov
Phone: 1-800-438-5383

National Diabetes Information Clearinghouse
The National Diabetes Information Clearinghouse (NDIC) was established in 1978 to increase knowledge and understanding about diabetes among patients, health care professionals, and the general public. To carry out this mission, NDIC works closely with NIDDK's Diabetes Research and Training Centers; the National Diabetes Education Program (NDEP); professional, patient, and voluntary associations; government agencies; and state health departments to identify and respond to informational needs about diabetes and its management.

Website: http://diabetes.niddk.nih.gov/index.htm
Phone: 1-800-860-8747

PUBLICATIONS FOR PEOPLE WITH DIABETES

Diabetes Health
www.diabeteshealth.com
Published continuously for 14 years, *Diabetes Health* magazine provides objective, sometimes controversial, but always balanced articles about living with diabetes. Consumers and medical professionals alike recognize the value of this niche magazine that treads where no other is willing to go.

Diabetes Forecast
www.diabetes.org/diabetes-forecast.jsp
Each month, nearly 4.4 million readers turn to *Diabetes Forecast* for the latest and best information on diabetes research and treatment and for practical tips on day-to-day coping with diabetes.

Diabetes Self-Management
www.diabetesselfmanagement.com
Diabetes Self-Management offers up-to-date, practical "how-to" information on nutrition, exercise, new drugs, medical advances, self-help, and the many other topics people need to know about to stay healthy. Over the last eight years alone, the articles and series in *Diabetes Self-Management* have captured 191 awards at the annual National Health Information Awards, more than any other diabetes magazine.

Diabetes Wellness News
www.diabeteswellness.net/wellness
Diabetes Wellness News is a monthly newsletter sent each month to members of the Diabetes Wellness Network and diabetes health professionals and clinics across the country. The newsletter contains news of recent advancements in

treatment, personal stories, and practical advice on all aspects of life with diabetes, encouraging self-management, and helping readers improve their blood glucose control.

BOOKS

There are so many wonderful books for people with diabetes that is difficult to choose just a few to recommend. I am going to give you some suggestions based on which ones I used as references for this book. The best source is the American Diabetes Association, and if you go to their online store at http://store.diabetes.org, you'll find so many wonderful books. These are some of my favorites.

The 101 Tips series
by various authors
These great little books give you exactly what they say: 101 tips for important subjects in diabetes self-care. There are over 10 individual titles in this series, and here's just a brief list of some of the titles: nutrition, raising healthy kids, pregnancy, medication, and weight loss.

American Diabetes Association Complete Guide to Diabetes, 4th Edition
by American Diabetes Association
This book is necessary for any person with diabetes. It'll give you all of the up-to-date knowledge and information you need to start educating yourself about diabetes and self-care.

Complete Guide to Carb Counting
by Hope Warshaw and Karmeen Kulkarni
Carb counting is one of the best tools for sticking with a meal plan, and these two wonderful educators and dietitians can give you the best information to begin.

Diabesity: The Obesity-Diabetes Epidemic that Threatens America—and What We Must Do to Stop It
by Francine Kaufman
Experts predict that more than one-third of American children born in 2000 will develop diabetes and that obesity is a major contributor. Inside Fran's book, you'll get a shocking look at this disease.

Diabetes: A Guide to Living Well, 4th Edition
by Gary Arsham and Ernest Lowe
Dr. Arsham is a diabetes educator and has spent many years teaching people how to live well with diabetes. This is a wonderful, inspiring book written by a man, a doctor, and an educator who just happens to have type 1 diabetes.

The Disaster Preparedness Guide for People with Diabetes
by the American Diabetes Association
This little booklet may not look like much, but it can help you get prepared for any kind of disaster that may occur in your area. Don't let yourself get caught off guard.

Guide to Healthy Restaurant Eating, 3rd Edition
by Hope Warshaw
This great little book gives you all of the nutritional data you'll need for eating out. It covers the menu items for more than 60 restaurant chains all over the nation.

Month of Meals series
by various authors
This cookbook series has pages that are split into three parts, one for breakfast, lunch, and dinner. Each part has a separate recipe on it, complete with nutritional information, so you don't have to get tired of eating the same

meals day after day. Instead, with these cookbooks, you can put together meal plans that are different and still meet your dietary goals.

The New Soul Food Cookbook for People with Diabetes, 2nd Edition
by Fabiola Demps Gaines and Roniece Weaver
Soul food used to be one of those foods that people had to cut out of their diets if they had diabetes. If you have this cookbook, you won't have to, and I think that's good enough reason to get this book for your kitchen.

COMPANIES THAT PROVIDE EDUCATIONAL MATERIALS

I have visited these sites many times before, but remember that the Internet changes quickly. Don't forget about the value of searching the Internet for diabetes information. I hope that the sites listed here will give you a good place to start. I think that you will enjoy them, and I know I was impressed by the materials you can find online. Enjoy!

Abbott
www.diabeteshealthconnection.com
This interesting website connects you to other websites about diabetes. It also will link you to Diabetes Control articles, which are a great resource for educational information and guidance. From this site, you can also reach these three sites:

www.diabetescontrolforlife.com
www.glucerna.com
www.abbottdiabetescare.com

Amylin
www.byetta.com
This is the website for the new drug Byetta (see chapter 2). Because it is a new drug, you might want to find out about it and how it is used differently from other medications for type 2 diabetes. The site has educational materials about diabetes, too.

Animas
www.animascorp.com
Animas makes insulin pumps. This website describes the concepts behind insulin pumps, discusses how and why they are used, and provides instructions for pump patients.

Bayer
www.bayercarediabetes.com
Bayer manufactures the Ascencia glucose meters, and this website discusses their meters, describes the use and care of these meters, and provides diabetes educational materials.

BD
www.bddiabetes.com
BD is best known for their syringes and needles. It was the first insulin syringe company. Their diabetes education materials are available on this site.

Eli Lilly Company
www.lillydiabetes.com
Learn more about insulin and managing your diabetes at this website. Eli Lilly will also send you lots of materials on diabetes self-management.

GlaxoSmithKline
www.gsk.com/yourhealth/diabetes.htm
www.avandia.com
These sites give you information about certain oral diabetes medications and have all kinds of diabetes educational materials that you can download or request by mail.

Insulet
www.myomnipod.com
Insulet makes a new kind of insulin pump, and this site offers educational materials about using pumps.

Lifescan
www.lifescan.com
This site will give you all kinds of information on Lifescan meters, including the very popular OneTouch. You will find information about computerizing your results and linking with their website. Interesting patient information is also available.

Medtronic
www.medtronic.com/patients/diabetes.html
This site discusses insulin pumps and continuous glucose monitoring. The latter is a fairly new concept, so you might want to check it out.

Merck
www.merck.com/consumer
This site describes Merck's medications and has information on its patient assistance program.

Novo Nordisk

www.novonordisk-us.com
This site describes Novo Nordisk products and provides educational materials. The website also discusses the changing health care system in the U.S. It gives great advice as to how we can make it better and use it properly.

Pfizer

www.exubera.com
www.pfizer.com
This site will tell you all about inhaled insulin and how it is being used throughout the country. It contains all kinds of educational materials. Take a look.

Roche

www.accu-chek.com
www.disetronic-usa.com
www.health-kiosk.ch/start_diabetes.htm
These sites all discuss the Roche Accu-Chek meters and Spirit insulin pumps. There are all kinds of educational materials available, and you can sign up for e-mails from the company to be informed when new developments arise.

Sanofi-Aventis

www.diabeteswatch.com
www.goinsulin.com
These sites discuss insulin administration and address the fears and concerns that arise when a person starts insulin.

Smiths Medical

www.cozmore.com

This site is about the CozMore insulin pump. It gives you educational materials and links you to several other sites that can be helpful.

Takeda

www.actos.com

This site describes the oral medication Actos (pioglitazone). It is in English and Spanish and has educational materials in both languages as well. This is a great new development!

Index

insulin (*continued*)
  resistance, 29, 43, 83
  therapy, 31–32, 37–39,
    41–55
  types, 45–48, 53
insurance, 37, 129, 132–133,
  151, 179–188, 192, 194
intercourse, 171–176
intermediate insulin, 45–47
iodine, radioactive, 42
islet cells, 28
isolation, 6–9

K

Kaufman, Fran,
  Diabesity, 149–150, 245
  neuropathy, 213
ketones, 138–139, 153,
  202–203, 207
kidney, 41, 82–83, 201,
  208–210, 217–218
Kruger, Davida, *Diabetes Travel
  Guide*, 171
Kübler-Ross, Elisabeth, *On Death
  and Dying*, 6–7
Kulkarni, Karmeen, *Complete
  Guide to Carb Counting*, 80,
  244
Kumamato Study, 200

L

labels, 79, 81, 86, 92–93
laboratory tests, 139–140,
  179–180
lactose, 74–75
lancing devices, 124–128
language, 168

Lantis insulin, 42
LDL (low-density lipoprotein),
  86, 210
letters, 20–26
Levitra, 175–176
levulose, 75
Lion's Club, 190
lipids, 57, 73
liquor, 165–167
liver, 41, 43
log, 70–71, 117–122, 135–136,
  158–159, 179–181
long-acting insulin, 48
low-density lipoprotein (LDL),
  86, 210

M

macroalbuminuria, 208
main courses, 98, 100–109
meal planning, 35, 37, 61–72,
  77–87
Medicaid, 133, 178, 195
medical ethics, 32
MedicAlert bracelet, 152, 169
Medicare, 133, 151, 178, 181,
  188, 190–195, 216
*Medicare Coverage of Diabetes
  Supplies & Services*
  (Medicare), 194
medications, *See names of* individual medications
  additional, 56–59
  administering, 49–56
  alcohol and, 166
  diabetes management, 31–37
  diabetes treatment, 113
  effect of, 37–40
  erectile dysfunction, 175–176
  hyperglycemia and, 202

Other Titles Available from the American Diabetes Association

Diabetes Meal Planning Made Easy, 3rd Edition

by Hope S. Warshaw, MMSc, RD, CDE, BC-ADM

Let expert Hope Warshaw show you how to change unhealthy eating habits while continuing to enjoy the foods you love! This book serves up techniques for changing your eating habits over time so that changes you make are the ones that last for life!

Order no. 4706-03; Price $14.95

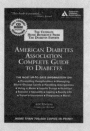

American Diabetes Association Complete Guide to Diabetes, 4th Edition

by American Diabetes Association

Have all the tips and information on diabetes that you need close at hand. The world's largest collection of diabetes self-care tips, techniques, and tricks for solving diabetes-related problems is back in its fourth edition, and it's bigger and better than ever before.

Order no. 4809-04; Price $29.95

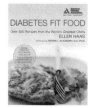

Diabetes Fit Food

by Ellen Haas

Put tasteless, boring recipes in the past with this new diabetes cookbook from healthy-eating expert Ellen Haas. She has compiled amazing, healthy recipes from some of America's best celebrity chefs, including Todd English, Alice Waters, and others. Finally, you can make sensible, healthy eating taste like it comes from a five-star restaurant.

Order no. 4661-014; Price $16.95

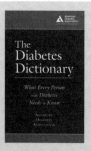

The Diabetes Dictionary

by American Diabetes Association

Diabetes can be a complicated disease; so to stay healthy, you need to understand the constantly growing vocabulary of diabetes research and treatment. *The Diabetes Dictionary* gives you the straightforward definitions of diabetes terms and concepts that you need to successfully manage your disease. With more than 500 entries, this pocket-size book is an indispensable resource for every person with diabetes.

Order no. 5020-01; Price $5.95

To order these and other great American Diabetes Association titles, call 1-800-232-6733 or visit http://store.diabetes.org. American Diabetes Association titles are also available in bookstores nationwide.

About the
American Diabetes Association

The American Diabetes Association is the nation's leading voluntary health organization supporting diabetes research, information, and advocacy. Its mission is to prevent and cure diabetes and to improve the lives of all people affected by diabetes. The American Diabetes Association is the leading publisher of comprehensive diabetes information. Its huge library of practical and authoritative books for people with diabetes covers every aspect of self-care—cooking and nutrition, fitness, weight control, medications, complications, emotional issues, and general self-care.

To order American Diabetes Association books: Call 1-800-232-6733 or log on to *http://store.diabetes.org*

To join the American Diabetes Association: Call 1-800-806-7801 or log on to *www.diabetes.org/membership*

For more information about diabetes or ADA programs and services: Call 1-800-342-2383. E-mail: AskADA@diabetes.org or log on to *www.diabetes.org*

To locate an ADA/NCQA Recognized Provider of quality diabetes care in your area: *www.ncqa.org/dprp*

To find an ADA Recognized Education Program in your area: Call 1-800-342-2383. *www.diabetes.org/for-health-professionals-and-scientists/recognition/edrecognition.jsp*

To join the fight to increase funding for diabetes research, end discrimination, and improve insurance coverage: Call 1-800-342-2383. *www.diabetes.org/advocacy-and-legalresources/advocacy.jsp*

To find out how you can get involved with the programs in your community: Call 1-800-342-2383. See below for program Web addresses.

American Diabetes Month: educational activities aimed at those diagnosed with diabetes—month of November. *www.diabetes.org/communityprograms-and-localevents/ americandiabetesmonth.jsp*

American Diabetes Alert: annual public awareness campaign to find the undiagnosed—held the fourth Tuesday in March. *www.diabetes.org/communityprograms-and-localevents/ americandiabetesalert.jsp*

American Diabetes Association Latino Initiative: diabetes awareness program targeted to the Latino community. *www.diabetes.org/communityprograms-and-localevents/latinos.jsp*

African American Program: diabetes awareness program targeted to the African American community. *www.diabetes.org/ communityprograms-and-localevents/africanamericans.jsp*

Awakening the Spirit: Pathways to Diabetes Prevention & Control: diabetes awareness program targeted to the Native American community. *www.diabetes.org/communityprograms-and-localevents/nativeamericans.jsp*

To find out about an important research project regarding type 2 diabetes: *www.diabetes.org/diabetes-research/research-home.jsp*

To obtain information on making a planned gift or charitable bequest: Call 1-888-700-7029. *www.wpg.cc/stl/CDA/homepage/ 1,1006,509,00.html*

To make a donation or memorial contribution: Call 1-800-342-2383. *www.diabetes.org/support-the-cause/make-a-donation.jsp*

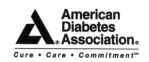